# Let Them In

## 30 Years of Secret Experiences

Karen Cavalli

# DEDICATION

To Bob V. who provided guidance and direction on this project; to Renee, John C. and Lynn E.F.H, my Virginia dear ones.

To Tom, my everything.

# CONTENTS

# INTRODUCTION

This book is relatively short, though it doesn't lend itself to skimming or speed-reading. The topic is intense. I'm steeped in it, but you may not be. Approach each of the book's four chapters as though it were tapas—those small, savory dishes best enjoyed slowly.

If you have had what I call secret experiences, what may also be called encounters with anomalous beings, the extraordinary or the paranormal, I believe you can integrate them and their effects into your life. I had over 30 years of secret experiences. They started when I was 10 and lasted into my 40s. I kept that life strand or life stream hidden for all those years and beyond, into my 50s. I had two life streams, Girl in Life Stream One, and Girl in Life Stream Two. Girl in Life Stream One was smart and outgoing with a talent for music and writing. Her potential careers were overshadowed by her anomaly career in Life Stream Two.[1] What if I had had guides? This book aspires to be a guide to anyone who is struggling to understand and integrate their secret experiences.

Whitley Strieber writes in *Transformation,* "It feels as if the best of my life has been lived in secret" (p. 113). Is the best part of your life hidden? If you wish to bring it out of hiding and weave it into the other strands of your life, this book may help.

Most of us don't have the option to apprentice to a tribal shaman in the US southwestern desert or Brazilian rain forest. Most of us are

---

[1] Courtesy of Craig Lang. the phrase "anomaly career" appears on page 6 of his article, "Close Encounters: The More We Learn, the Less We Know."

tied to things in this world including jobs we must stay at in order to keep money coming in. Popular notions would say you create your own reality. I believe this generally, but temper it with the awareness that we exist alongside those abilities in everyone else; that's a lot of power knocking up against power. Too, serving up new realities takes time. The beings you encounter in secret experiences have a definite reality but one that is not yet reflected in our current culture. You must deal with the effects of the secret experiences without a lot of support from the waking culture. This is true overtly, since it's rare to meet with belief when you tell others of a secret experience, and covertly. The reality of those who populate secret experiences has yet to infiltrate our culture to the degree that their symbols are reflected in ours.

You could take my journey and spend 40 years bridging the two worlds; or maybe I could help you get there faster. Besides, I'd welcome the company.

# 1 MY SECRET EXPERIENCES

My experiences began in 1964 in Tacoma, Washington. My dad was stationed on an aircraft carrier off the coast of Vietnam and ran air operations. He was considered "blue water Navy," too far from the coast to be affected by dioxin, found in the herbicide Agent Orange sprayed over the jungles of Vietnam. He would die many years later of lymphoma, the cancer associated with dioxin exposure.

In 1964, while my dad was on ship, we were living in a neighborhood in Tacoma that bordered a field. On the opposite side of the field ran a creek. In 1964 or '65 UFOs were sighted in Tacoma. I was six years old. I recall curfews in our neighborhood as a result, and lying in bed trying to go to sleep on one of those summer evenings. I recall a shadow passing my bedroom window. I sleep walked that year, going to stand on the front step of our house and calling for my mother. Either my mom would wake and bring me back inside or a neighbor would, waking my mom in the process. My mom pushed a recliner in front of the door to prevent me from opening it; in my sleep I pushed it away to resume calling for my mother on the front step. This is what my mother told me; I don't have any memory of it.

My dad came home, and the military moved us next to Yuma, Arizona, another quiet time for me secret experience-wise. We lived first in El Pueblocito then moved into base housing at the Yuma Marine Corps Air Station, where my dad also worked, still in air traffic control.

My father left the military a few years later to begin a career in banking, transporting our family from the camaraderie of military base life and a new neighborhood every two years—Tsuruma, Japan; Olathe, Kansas; Blackbush, England; Brunswick, Georgia; Tacoma, Washington; Yuma, Arizona—to a place of great beauty and isolation. My secret experiences began here in 1968, in my bedroom in our house set among the pines and birch of the northern Minnesota woods.

As I lay in bed, trying to fall asleep, the deep woods not far from my bedroom window, my head filled with what seemed like many radio stations coming in on the same frequency—words, snippets of sentences, overlapping conversations. I caught a phrase here and there, and occasionally heard my name being spoken.

Then the dreams began: aliens came calling, and the first one they sent looked like a human boy. His name was Eric. I dreamed of Eric taking me and another woman on tours of different planets. I don't recall anything specific about the planets or the inhabitants. Eric's spaceship looked like the model George Jetson operates – a saucer with a round, clear top so the riders can see out.

During these years I began having a kind of dream that persisted into about my 20s. I sat silently with a solitary alien as it transmitted knowledge telepathically into my mind. I recall there were at least two types of extraterrestrials, but only remember one which seemed to be made of black and red metal.

One of these early years in Minnesota my sister Annette and I were rained on by frogs on a cold Christmas walk in a snowy field near our house. A swarm of frogs seemed to fly up from under the snow and begin pelting us. I recall the thwacking sound as they landed against my winter jacket. We screamed and laughed hysterically, falling over ourselves in our scramble to get back to the lighted house about 500 yards ahead of us.

A memory during these years, the early to mid-70s: I was babysitting my brother and two younger sisters. My older sister Chrissy had left home for college. It was summer, and we stood outside staring up at the night sky, transfixed: against the dark sky diffuse white light flowed back and forth, ebbing and flowing like ocean waves, taking shapes. I recall calling the nearest airport (Brainerd) to report this. The next morning a red mist covered everything near our house.

At about this same time, in the early to mid-1970s, my parents saw what they describe as "strange lights" coming home one night from a rare dinner out. I didn't learn of their experience until many years later, in the late 1990s when I was working on recording all my experiences with unusual phenomena. At the time of my parents' sighting, much of the area where we lived was covered in forest, including the area near our house and the highway leading to it. They were on that highway when they saw the strange lights. My dad told me how they drove around the dark, empty roads near our house trying to locate the source. They saw what appeared to be a huge light source hovering close to the ground in the woods a ways off the highway.

In May of 1976 when I was 17 and a few months away from graduating high school a Man in Black paid me a visit.

I'd fallen asleep one spring night after watching television in our house's downstairs TV room. At that time and in that part of the country, television stations signed off at midnight. The overhead light and the static from the pixilated television screen woke me.

I experienced a moment of disorientation as my eyes opened to see a man's wool-trousered knees. I lay on my side and the knees were directly in front of me at eye level. My gaze traveled slowly up the trouser legs, as though this was a mannequin standing in front of me, and I took in the black briefcase, the skinny black tie, the matching black suit jacket (the wool fabric wasn't solid black—there were tiny flecks of another color, the same kind of variety you see in a good wool suit).

Up until that point, it was as though I were viewing an inanimate object, part of the landscape of such objects in my view: monkey wood coffee table, brown braided rug, paneled walls. Then my eyes reached his face and the terrible numbing fright began.

His eyes glowed green. He sported a bowler. His head was tilted, as though better to gaze at me, and he grinned. I could feel my eyes, muscles and limbs lock in fear, as I lay like a stunned animal, mesmerized by his eyes.

I couldn't rise from the couch, but I knew if I started screaming, my parents would come eventually. I fought the paralysis and raised my hands to eyes to hide him from my sight and started screaming.

I screamed a long time. When finally I heard my mom and dad stumbling down the stairs, that broke the spell. I vaulted over the couch and into my father's arms.

My parents settled me on the couch in the upstairs living room. I sat there stunned with fear and asked my dad to search the house. He agreed, and only many years later did he confess he actually had not searched the house.

At that point I'd been living in the deep woods for about seven years, with one summer at 16 spent in Renton, Washington, with a cousin and her family. After graduation from high school, I was on fire with movement, and for the next several years ping-ponged back and from the west and east coasts (with a brief interlude at the University of Minnesota where I saw my first demon; for details see "Secret Experiences—Feelings and Responses'") then settled in the Tidewater region of Virginia.

For the next six years, from 1978 to 1984, the dreams didn't occur as often. When they did, they were as benign as those in the early years. Eric returned and we took more rides around the galaxy. I started seeing people in my peripheral vision, people who were not there, and had accompanying nightmares that I could see what others could not.

During the last several months I lived in Norfolk, I began hearing angels singing. Or at least that's what I identified it as. It was definitely singing, and the voices sounded celestial, of the heavens. It was a chorus of voices, mostly high, and with a thin rather than full sound. It was a beautiful sound. It occurred randomly and didn't seem associated to any particular setting, event or people.

Activity started up again in 1986, a year before I finished graduate school at the University of Alabama in Tuscaloosa. In one dream of March that year the earth was taken over by beings from another planet. From my journal that March: "They were tall, like Alice Goon, and wore dark robes that hooded their faces. The world was completely changed. Four of them were gardening, and each wore plastic plaid aprons to protect their robes."

From another journal entry that same month:

> I took hold of a rope of soft, tattered cotton and swung up into the heavens. I saw the goddess and she was beautiful, naked, and lying in the clouds. The goddess was showing me and another person what to do, but we couldn't get it. Then something happened to the goddess. She was dying and we couldn't save her. She fell into a cloud-puddle and died.
>
> Scorpions immediately began crawling over her.

I graduated in the spring of 1987 and returned to the Tidewater area of Virginia. Big mistake. I thought I was returning to the same group of friends who had been like a family to me before I left. I did return to those same people, but everyone had moved on. I did have family there, my sister Chrissy, and she helped me get settled.

However, she too had formed new relationships, and I felt as though I were the odd one out. It even seemed that all the people I'd loved were turning away from me.

I got a job as an Editorial Assistant at what was then the *Virginian-Pilot / Ledger-Star*, the state's largest newspaper. I did alright but felt numb and lost from the loss of my old circle.

On August 15, 1987, I dreamed that all dreams were interrupted, and we were called up into the goddess ship. From my journal:

> We were held in the honey-combed hold while three
>
> goddesses stood at the front. They wore gowns and jewels.
>
> After some time of us looking at them and them looking at
>
> us, they returned us to our dreams.

Once returned to our dreams we all compared our experiences in the goddess ship.

This was the last dream I had for a long time, a long time for me, anyway – about four months.

The next day – it was that abrupt – I changed as though I'd become a creature not meant for the physics of this planet. I had episodes of invisibility that continued into the mid-1990s. People often could not see me or hear me speak. At one point as I sat in my car and waited at a red light near Old Dominion University in Norfolk, Virginia, pedestrians gathered near my car, peering in and saying, "There's no one driving that car."

At times people and things appeared to me as columns of shimmering energy. I seemed to lose my place on the time continuum, shifting a bit ahead or back, my sense registering the sounds and sights of those future and past times. While talking with people I heard conversations they'd had earlier with someone else as well as the audio of events that had occurred in their past, a kind of aural clairvoyance in reverse. I heard my dad eating popcorn as we talked on the phone, and he told me wasn't eating popcorn at that moment but had been earlier. If I dropped something such as a pen, I heard the air waves splitting as the pen fell through them in slow motion. This continued into the mid-1990s.

I dreamed of people from another dimension trapping me and a friend in my parents' home, refusing to let us go until they said to us what they'd come to say. I first saw an old man in my peripheral vision. I didn't pay attention because in waking life I often saw people in my peripheral vision. Then he came in front of me as an actual person and following him were an old woman and a young woman with dark hair and a white tail. In the dream I knew they were people or ghosts from the underworld. The woman with the dark hair and a white tail told me that when we see people in our peripheral vision we are seeing people from other dimensions, people who move alongside us all the time but most people can't see. She also told me that this ability comes from our mothers. Then we let these other-dimensional beings hang out with us like anyone from our dimension. We showed them how to turn on lights and play the radio. Eventually my friend and I left.

I saw bronze giants on the side of the road as I drove from Suffolk to Smithfield, Virginia.

Starting in November of 1987 and continuing through February of 1988 I had a series of dreams in which I underwent initiation to become a witch.

I had another dream of sitting with a creature while it transmitted information telepathically to me. This was the only time I remembered the exact words. "Get to know the Lizard Men of revelations; we need more of their kind."

Is that revelations with a big R or little r? I figured I'd play along, give in, accept the mission. I started with the biblical Revelations, and found no mention of lizard men. I tried meditating on lizard men. I just started thinking about them, sitting in my Norfolk, Virginia, attic room I rented in the house of a friend's mother. This was in June of 1988. I'd left my job at the newspaper. I planned to pick strawberries at the break of dawn as a way to make money. A friend had connected me with a writer for *Reader's Digest*, a married man in his 40s. My friend was hoping to help me get published. The *Reader's Digest* writer was hoping to get laid. Well, weren't we all? Not me with a married friend of a friend.

A story grew as I fell into a state of half sleep, half wakefulness. I was with someone, a person whose sex was unclear. This person was part of a network that helped hide wise reptiles in walls within walls in houses. She/he pulled down the walls, and there they were, human-sized reptiles with the ability to speak. One particularly ugly reptile placed the "scale of truth" around my neck. The reptiles scared me.

The next day I heard news reports of sightings of a large lizard man in the woods of South Carolina.

Fabulous. I couldn't fix my broken-down life but I could summon lizard men into our dimension. There's a skill worth noting on a resume!

I couldn't get myself out of bed in time to pick strawberries in the fields outside Norfolk and instead started working temp office jobs.

I started dating a man who lived in southern Maryland. He lived with his parents. I'd known him and his family for a while through a friend who had dated his brother. I spent a few weekends visiting him and his parents. His mother encouraged me to apply for jobs in their area. I took a position coordinating state writing exam preparation at nearby LaPlata High School in Maryland. I was working alongside licensed teachers. I had no educational background in education, no license. I had a masters in writing. Several got sour looks on their face when they had to be near me. Several would not speak to me, even to answer my questions. I got a taste of what teaching ninth graders was like, and became friends with two of the teachers, a fellow English teacher and the Art teacher, and Kate the librarian.

In December of 1988 I dreamed our entire planet was being taken over by aliens. I saw them once, and then only in shadow. They were long and thin beings.

For several months in the spring of 1989 I heard a clear voice within me introduce itself and offer advice. When I asked what it was, it responded, "an Endoform." One night it spoke excitedly and with jubilance; the next morning it was gone. I learned later that day one of the teachers, a friendly acquaintance, had given birth the night before.

In April of 1989, while still in Maryland, I dreamed an enormous flying saucer landed near my parents' house in Minnesota, where they still lived in the deep woods. I saw the saucer close up. It had blinking, colored lights, a silver, curved underbelly and shapes moving around inside. The next morning (in the dream) it was disguised as a military base.

That spring I broke up with the man I'd been seeing, and when my basement apartment flooded, had no one to call for help but one of the vice principals. I also called my sister Chrissy, who, after I explained the situation, said I could stay with her in the house she rented in Chuckatuck, Virginia, while I finished grading final exams.

In June 1989, I dreamed I was high up and watching an ancient battle between a human and a reptile man. They were enemies yet friends. Reptile man called a truce and leaned heavily against a tree. The other man was gone, and the reptile man lay on a plot of grass with strange white markings. The earth began to shake then the earth swallowed up the reptile man's inert form.

After the school year ended I packed up my things and my cat Margaret in my yellow Datsun and drove 1500 miles to my parents' house in the deep woods.

That fall I woke in the dark to loud knocking, three rhythmic knocks, as though knuckles were rapping on a door outside my bedroom window. There was no one there.

I had several dreams in which the aliens used my physical body as a medium for their transformation into our dimension. In one dream they tried to use the voice boxes of me and my older sister to vocalize their message. I don't know what the message was; according to my recollection of the dreams, the experiment was not successful. My sister and I gurgled a lot, bent double from the force of their message as it poured down into us from the sky, a silvery, glittery stream of stars.

My dream journal entry in October of 1989 reads, "First, space aliens landed. They and I were pleasantly involved." The November 1989 entry reads, "Space invaders were on our planet, in our neighborhood. We humans were not supposed to be too visible and so we sneaked around from building to building after dark."

In January of 1990 I moved to Minneapolis and took a part-time job in arts administration at what at that time was known as The World Theatre (now The Fitzgerald), from which Garrison Keillor broadcast "A Prairie Home Companion." I became friends with some of my coworkers and started to build a life.

From my dream journal, January 1990:

> I met a person – sex and age unclear – and this being sat in
> my bedroom and we talked. This being was not from this
> planet. The being told me its name – I had a hard time with it
> in the dream, as I did when I woke and recorded the dream.
> Beattakuka or something like that. I asked Be if when in
> previous dreams I'd visited other planets, had I really done

so? And Be nodded knowingly, began to speak and
something interrupted.

April 1990: "The man in black was back, and I was trying to
convince my friends."

Two dreams from October 1990:

At the end of a dream I and my husband [my dream husband,
I guess, since I didn't have one in waking life] saw what
looked like a giant spacecraft hovering above us, but it was
only a reflection.

At the end of the dream the moon landed in the front yard
and was lighted in spots like a city. Smaller satellite moons
spiraled off and toward me. I ran, scared, to the bedroom,
and someone told me it was only a reflection.

Two other dreams during this time: in the first, I was transported
out of my bedroom in the house I rented in the Seward
neighborhood of Minneapolis, on my way to a waiting ship. I don't
remember getting there but remember the method of transport: I lay
prone on something flat, stretcher-like, and was bound in white cloth
like a swaddled child. In the dream I thought, "Is this how I
developed claustrophobia?" I seemed to be of two minds in the
dream, the dreamer mind and my waking, conscious mind asking that
question. I have had claustrophobia in waking life since I was a child,
severe enough to stop a small plane before take-off, saying to the
flight attendant, "I have to get off. I have claustrophobia. I can't do
this" (in the days before this would get you arrested) and to have to
ask to be taken out of a sweat lodge mid-ritual in Tuscaloosa,

Alabama. In the second, several of us humans were made to watch films of the moon exploding and other cataclysmic planetary events.

In the early 1990s welts began forming all over my body and my uterus went crazy, knocking against the inside of my body like something trying to get out. A change in temperature or light would cause the welts to rise, winding like a snake all over my body. The only thing that offered relief was the one thing I was allergic to at that time – a certain type of antihistamine. I saw a doctor at the University of Minnesota for my rocking uterus who said "I've never seen anything like it." I saw a chiropractor in St. Paul, and she diagnosed "burned-out adrenals" and prescribed a course of action, including changes to diet and adding supplements. It worked.

During this time I was still trying to figure out how to work at a job that brought in enough to pay the bills but freed me mentally to continue writing. I wrote primarily short fiction, and began to get published and win awards. An acquaintance asked me if I'd co-write a book on AIDS with him, and that resulted in my first book publication, followed by a second on girls' development for the same publisher (Lerner Publications). Both books won awards. Due to the AIDS book, an organization invited me on a trip to Africa, on which I'd be joined by others in the AIDS field. I didn't have the money to join the trip.

I was temping again. I got up at 3 am to write fiction. I dreamed of my dead grandparents, my mother's parents, who in the after-world had divorced. My grandmother did not speak but guided me to safe places. My grandfather had remarried and had grown out his hair past his shoulders, donned knee-high fringed boots and in one dream provided specific information about American Vaudeville for a story I was working on, letting me know I had the name of one of the stage performers wrong and giving me the correct name. When my cat Margaret died she often joined my grandparents in these dream visits.

I kept my writing routine while writing the AIDS book, rising at 3 am to write. After writing I'd hop a bus to downtown Minneapolis to get to my temp job by 8 am. Most nights I was in bed by 7 p.m. to start it all over again at 3 am. Six hours of sleep wasn't enough for me, but I couldn't see where else to pare things down. I gained weight and cut my hair into a short bob. White streaks started to appear, and the rest of my dark blonde hair turned the color of nails. Wearing high heels of even modest height (one to two inches) hobbled me, and I bought a pair of Red Wing Postman black lace-ups, the only shoes I could wear for a long time. There was nothing supernatural about any of this; just aging without the help of hair coloring and better shoe sense.

I developed a class for the University of Minnesota's Compleat Scholar Program: "In the Land Between Heartbeats: Stories of Descent." I offered literature and writing exercises as a way of understanding experiences that pull you out of life. I included any experience on a broad continuum of experiences, from the sadly common (loss, rejection, grief) to the extraordinary (other-worldly beings and experiences). Even those common or at least known experiences can knock many people out of their orbit and render them stunned. The more unusual or extraordinary experiences seem to have the power to expel people from their lives. What do you do when you aren't where you used to be but aren't yet where you're going? I intended the course to help people answer this by integrating their experience through literature that spoke to it and writing exercises. I also had a secret intent: find some pals on this crazy journey.

And I found them. For four years in a row the class filled, and in some cases the class members and I continued meeting after the course ended.

In one dream during this period, the aliens gave me an instrument a long tube like the Aborigine's didgeridoo. I blew on one end, and tiny white feathers came out the other, and this allowed the aliens to metamorphose from their dimension into the physicality of ours. The morning after this dream, I woke to find tiny white feathers littered about my dining room. My response was to be stunned. I just stood there, immobilized, unable to process anything. The shock blunted any intelligence I had. Mechanically, I vacuumed up the feathers, placed the vacuum cleaner bag in the trash at the curb, and when I returned home from work later that day, I put away the empty trash can.

I dreamed the aliens rolled back the scrim of the sky to show me their handiwork – a new universe they'd created, right alongside ours.

About that time a friend of mine's 18-year-old son got a job in IT or Information Technology making more than I was making. Often I read of people who did what they loved and the money followed. I thought this meant money trailed them, like a cat after tuna, the power of doing what they loved attracting money. But I came to realize "follow" meant comes second . . . or third . . . or fourth; you get the picture. I was my sole source of money; I couldn't figure out how to have money without working to make it. And so I moved into technical IT support, troubleshooting mainframe and network issues, where demand for help was high. This was before outsourcing moved many of these jobs offshore, and the need in the US was great enough that companies would take people with a basic knowledge and aptitude and train them.

I was 39. I moved from technical support into knowledge management at a local software company. The sun was setting on my reproductive years; I loved it that I was finally getting to an age when people would stop assuming I had mating and reproduction on my mind. I took up yoga, lost 40 pounds and gained a half-inch in height. I started coloring my hair and got better shoe sense (though I held on to my Red Wing Postman's). My secret experiences dwindled to only the occasional dream of the aliens finding their way among us on our planet. At 42 I met Tom who I would marry five years later.

My mom passed away in 2002, and my dad in 2011. The summer after my dad's passing I shredded my journals, 40 years' worth.

In the fall of that year I discovered I'd excerpted dreams from those journals and placed them in the file with the materials from the "In the Land Between Heartbeats" course. I also re-discovered the electronic copy of a recounting of all my experiences, intended for a book, from about 2002.

In 2011 a business acquaintance recommended me for the Mrs. Minnesota-America pageant. After some preliminary qualifying steps, I became the official Mrs. Savage, representing the City of Savage in the upcoming March 2012 pageant.

After a job lay-off in November 2011 I met a small business adviser through my hair stylist who offered suggestions on what to do with this writing, and you are reading the result.

In 2011 I added Reiki to my yoga practice. I'm certified at the second level, and mostly practice on myself, family and critters but also offer stealth Reiki when someone needs immediate comfort.

About this time I dreamed I woke up inside a dream to see my dad behind a line of trees. I could feel I was using a different kind of sight – I felt it in my eyeballs. I could also see there was a grey film or veil over my vision. I was about 150 yards opposite my dad, standing on the edge of a field that bordered the grassy dip in the land between us. I felt it was understood I could not go any closer to dad, and he could not come closer to me. He was receptive, standing, smiling. He looked like he did about a year before he passed, when he was still in relatively stable health, having recovered from various illnesses. His clothes hung on him as they did at that time, having lost weight from illness. He wore trousers, a collared shirt, one of those light-weight jackets he always wore. He rocked from foot to foot, as though ready to jump behind a tree to get out of sight.

Later I would learn this is considered a lucid dream, where you wake up inside the dream. The idea is that you are able to have more control over the dream's outcome and perhaps over your waking life as well. There are techniques to employ that supposedly increase one's ability to have lucid dreams.

# 2 FEELINGS AND RESPONSES

Many of us who have had secret experiences get stuck in the aftermath of responses to the emotional and sometimes physical trauma. Secret experiences can wreck you—mind, body, feelings, spirit. The effects may occur on a scale, from low to high intensity. No matter where the effects may fall, understanding what is common to feel emotionally and physically may help to integrate the experience. Getting a glimpse of how secret experiences might change you can provide meaning and help you to grow from the experience.

In my own experiences I felt shaken and without inner resources. For most of my years of these experiences I had no one around me who could help me address the nature of the experiences head-on. I often felt overcome emotionally. I compartmentalized the experiences, categorizing them in my mind as only dreams or something imagined. I did this as long as I could, until the experiences and their effects left the dream realm and entered my waking life. Ultimately I found that bringing secret experiences into the light and allowing them to take on a greater sense of reality can provide structure and context for integrating these baffling experiences into everyday life.

In my most desolate of times, when it seemed I had lost all, my way, my home, those close to me, I found both kinship and allies through reading and writing. I took those solitary activities into the public, created a forum for people with similar experiences. I found sharing some of those experiences and hearing about others' reduced feelings of isolation. We were not alone, and we were not imagining things. For me that forum provided a secure base from which I could choose how I would live with my new reality.

I've observed two camps of secret experiencers: those whose lives stop at the onset of secret experiences, where they remain developmentally, and those who continue to engage with the world. This engagement may or may not look like a successful American life – career advancement, social standing, ability to procure material goods – but it fosters or perhaps ignites something in those individuals that allows them to keep forging ahead, day after day, taking on the demands of their daily lives and being remade by extraordinary encounters they didn't seek out. These are usually experienced as two separate streams of life. That was the case for me as I moved through 30 years of secret experiences. This is the case for other experiencers I've met, and a review of the literature tells me it is how many experiencers have managed the two ways of life calling to them.

There are exceptions. I recently met one. Paulette Salo, known as the angel artist, returned to her regular, waking life after encounters with angels in three near-death experiences (for more on her story visit http://angelsbypaulette.com/). Spaced over a period of 40 years, these encounters occurred about every 20 years at ages 20, 33 and 60. Only after the third encounter at 60 did Salo's angel journey to our physical world, appearing at Salo's hospital bedside to tell her her mission: to get people to talk to their angels. Salo also reports that all of her angel interactions have been pleasant, another exception to secret experiences of my own and those of others I've collected (personal communication, January 2014).

This section offers kinship and allies in the form of others' stories, including mine, to reduce anxiety and provide a base of support to give you options: to integrate the streams of your life; to go deeper into secret experiences; to become a student of extraordinary phenomenon; to become a watcher of your own life and perhaps discover your own meaning for your experiences; to do nothing; to engage less with the world; to engage more with the world; to find new allies; to be of service to those baffled, unnerved or shattered by their secret experiences; to be a voice for these experiences; perhaps to relax into whatever's happening without judgment or plans to turn it into vocation or commerce.

I would recommend that the first work of literature you read is Dr. Don Donderi's book, *UFOs, ETs and Alien Abductions: A Scientist Looks at the Evidence*, published in 2013. A scientist and former academic, he assembles and reviews the evidence indicating we are being visited by extraterrestrials and concludes, simply and coolly, that we are. The new lens that Donderi provides changed everything for me. All elements of doubt clouding my intellectual conception of what I've experienced faded away, and with that emerged a different way of viewing my life. I felt respect for that secret life where before I felt shame.

Donderi's book focuses on the evidence that extraterrestrials are visiting us, and therefore on alien abductions, one of the eight types of secret experiences I've defined. Of the eight, alien abductions are probably the one written most about. I've experienced seven of the eight, though encounters with extraterrestrials predominate.

See Appendix B for a matrix describing the emotions and bodily sensations that may accompany the eight types of secret experiences. The matrix is based on my experiences along with those of individuals I've come in contact with over the past 20 years through meetings and teaching on related topics. The main sections that follow here reference these effects and experiences as well as those that have been documented by others.

### Interrupted sleep and extreme fear

Physically, I experienced insomnia as a result of interrupted sleep for most of my 30 years of encounters with sentient beings not of a type known to our current reality. I woke from each dream as though it were a nightmare, even the dreams with the boyish Eric and his Jetson-style spaceship. The later information-transmission sessions, so oddly uneventful—just me and a machine-like alien facing each other as we sat at a table, left me terrified and breathless. I'd wake in the early morning hours, usually at 3 am, my heart thudding, nerves screaming with red alerts. I rarely went back to sleep, and for some reason told no one, not even my older sister with whom I shared a room. (Apparently my bolting awake never woke her.) I could not calm myself. I lay there vibrating with fear yet was physically still, a passivity similar to that which I exhibited in the dreams.

That insomniac rhythm stayed with me for many years, and only in my early 40s, when the frequency of the dreams and experiences began to taper off, did I again sleep through the night (and, coincidentally, gained half an inch in height). Tom, now my husband, was in my life at this point, and perhaps his presence, like a talisman, warded off the secret experiences.

## Guilt and atonement

I felt guilty most of the time. To atone, I went to work. I took my first job at 10 years old, working in the grade-school cafeteria in exchange for free lunches. I stood stationed behind a large, aluminum trash can, wearing an apron and a hair net, holding a spatula, while my fellow fifth and sixth graders sat at long tables and ate their lunch. As my classmates exited they handed me their trays, and I scraped their uneaten food into the trash. I also worked the food line, dishing up that day's lunch alongside the adult cafeteria workers. Our one-eyed manager wore a white food-service dress and thick-soled white shoes, and secured her black hair under the requisite hair net. When I couldn't stop coughing during bouts of bronchitis she fed me sugar as I stood next to her in the food line.

According to Alice Bryant and Linda Seebach in their book *Healing Shattered Reality: Understanding Contactee Trauma* experiencers feel guilt due to being chosen when others around them aren't (p. 57). I don't recall feeling chosen but definitely felt guilty.

## Feeling hunted

The emotions I experienced during my anomaly career were primarily a sense of strangeness, feeling watched and hunted; a strong desire to understand and the desire to answer the question, "Why me?"

I had two streams of life: average girl and strange and hunted girl. I developed an outward- and an inward-turning. At 10 I knew enough about astrology to win a television in a contest advertised on the back of a cereal box. In my early teens I found a book on spell-casting and began practicing the art of intention. I believed in the plasticity of reality. In my senior year of high school I developed a crush on a long-haired Vietnam vet and substitute school bus driver. I'd visit him at his ramshackle little house near the iron ore mine hills and make out with him on his broken-down couch. He introduced me to books on black magic. I also started reading texts like John Woolman's books on Quakerism, yet at the same time I pored over *Seventeen* magazine's Dear Beauty Editor column, read Victoria Holt novels and fell in love with Donny Osmond.

I made average grades in school except for English and band where my grades were higher. I wrote well and had a talent for playing the clarinet such that I caught the attention of my grandfather, a former Vaudeville performer and musician, and my grade school and high school music teachers. On a visit from Kansas

City, Missouri, where my grandparents lived, my grandfather gave me clarinet lessons. Tall, bony, exacting, he held my wrist in a death grip when making a point. I attended band camp in Canada the summer before ninth grade. In high school my band teacher drove me each Monday after school to a music lesson with a professor of music at a state university about an hour away. Up until high school I had an average social life then that life, too, split into two streams: in social life stream one I lived the life of the average girl as a cheerleader and majorette. I had best friends in each grade, and up until my senior year we called each other every morning to find out what the other was wearing and talked about what boys we had crushes on. In social life stream two on weekends I joined older high school students for illicit beer drinking around fires in the iron ore mine hills.

## Development of an early-warning system and desire to be on the move

In life stream one I was a young woman of musical talent with a natural ability to practice repetitiously. In life stream two, I was developing an acute early-warning system, ready for surprise encounters, and frequently felt paranoid. I was often poised to go on Red Alert, with my inner point-man patrolling the periphery of my consciousness. It was as though some ongoing chain of encounters or confrontations was ongoing behind the scrim of regular, daily life, as though some part of me had its own life in another dimension.

In my last years of high school I often felt on fire with the need to move, a restlessness that stayed with me into my late 30s. I interpreted it as a strong intuition, since it seemed to take over my thoughts and actions when it compelled me to move on.

To paraphrase Whitley Strieber in *Transformation*, I came to feel the biggest part of my life was lived in secret (p. 113). Girl in Life-Stream One came to feel two-dimensional, and what promise she held in the world of light would materialize only for a short time, between lulls in my anomaly career.

## Ontological shock and feelings of falling apart

I was overwhelmed by ontological shock, or the shock of my entire world view being thrown into question, and feelings I was falling apart after three secret experiences. The first two times, at ages 17 and 18, were short-lived and were more about my ego or overriding personality falling apart. The third time was longer in duration and more intense in affect. What I knew to be "I" was obliterated, and with that a world beyond physics I knew opened up, and for a time I moved into it. More vibration than solid matter, I sometimes appeared invisible to others.

The visit from a Man in Black, described in the "My Secret Experiences" chapter, resulted in my first experience with feeling I was falling apart.

Because my family didn't speak of what had happened the next day, or any time soon after that, I felt that old, cold fright when I first spoke with Peter Rojcewicz in March of 1990. Rojcewicz, formerly a Professor of Mythology at Julliard, writes on the Men in Black or

MIB phenomenon, a variety of the extraordinary which existed and was being studied well before Hollywood discovered it.

Though Rojcewicz views MIB as archetypal, the questions he asked pointed at their possible physicality: did the Man in Black leave footprints on the braid rug? Did I scream long enough to allow him to run out of the house? If not, were there places downstairs where he could have hidden until it was safe to leave?

Earliest recorded sightings of and encounters with Men in Black date back to about 500 A.D. Their appearance has not changed much over the centuries: Black suit and tie, briefcase, often a fedora-style hat, the kind American men wore in the 1950s, though once in a great while they are seen sporting a bowler. Most commonly they travel in twos and threes, and their visit to unsuspecting humans frequently follows unreported UFO sightings by those people. Generally, the timing of the MIB's visit occurs shortly after the sighting and during the day or at least at hours when most people would answer the front door. Often they arrive in large, black late model cars, such as Oldsmobile's. Most who have been visited by MIB take them for humans, albeit strange, threatening ones. Their message is short and usually the same: forget what you saw and tell no one, or there will be trouble. In reports of contemporary encounters, those who receive their visits note their mechanical speech and gait, giving the impression they are either new to speech and the physical body or their human appearance is a deception and perhaps hiding a non-human being.

Rojcewicz' general take on the phenomenon is that it is tied to others which percipients experience as real but the general populace considers myth: The Irish Little People, for example. Rojcewicz adheres to the Jungian notion of archetypes, images and experiences that cross cultures and manifest in a number of ways but have a similar core expression or meaning.

In his research, Rojcewicz has talked with a number of people who have been visited by MIB. Though upsetting, the visits which take place in the common fashion described above don't appear to cause most individuals to radically change their lives or become permanently marred. However, Rojcewicz has spoken to one person who was so shattered after his visit from a Man in Black that he abruptly left what had been a mostly normal life—work, family, home—and disappeared into the Maine wilderness.

More common, notes Rojcewicz, is to simply be shocked.

The second time I fell apart was after watching a demon pull itself from under my college dorm-room bed. I was 18, a freshman during my brief time at the University of Minnesota, and had just crawled into bed after studying. The bedside light was on. Something caught my eye, and I leaned over the bed. A being with flayed skin and a slash for a mouth was pulling itself out from under my bed. I jerked back and sat in shock on the bed, my back against the door room wall. "Come and get me," I said to my parents when I called them the next day. And so they did, and returned me to the dark northern woods.

The third experience was a series of dreams over three nights culminating in the dream in which all dreams were interrupted and all dreamers were called up into the mother ship. Preceding that dream were these: I passed through seven gates in darkness, and on the next night dreamed I ate the full moon. On the third night, August 15, 1987, I dreamed the culminating dream: all dreamers were called up into the mother ship and held in the honey-combed hold while three goddesses stood at the front. Each stood on a dais and each wore a jewel-colored gown with matching jewels. They looked at us, and we looked at them. We dreamers stood, in a bit of shock, grouped in our honey combs, wearing whatever we'd gone to bed in. Each honey comb was lit with submerged light. After some time the goddesses returned us to our dreams. The following day I was gone from myself. It happened that quickly. In the weeks that followed I saw people as columns of light, saw bronze giants on the side of the road from Suffolk to Smithfield and experienced spontaneous invisibility confirmed by onlookers. Appearing invisible to others continued off and on into the 1990s along with a sub-atomic experience of reality: I could feel the invisible, vibrating strings that connected all things. When my dad was preparing to call me, I could feel it, the feeling coming to me on one of those vibrating strings.

I struggled through those first few weeks after the mother ship dream, often crying uncontrollably as I viscerally experienced the end of who I was. At the same time I seemed to be subject to new laws of physics and had nothing and no one to guide me in this. People once near and dear to me drifted away. Even the tarot would no longer speak to me.

The acute sensation that I was experiencing the end of who I was continued for several months. I felt lost to myself and the life I'd once had in the Tidewater region of Virginia. It seemed individuals once close to me withdrew. In case you're wondering did anyone in my family or my circle of friends notice I seemed to be falling apart a lot? If they did, no one said anything. Yes, I realize how strange that sounds, but that's how it was. Jean Shinoda Bolen writes in *Gods in Everyman* of those times when a complex overwhelms the personality and how people around you may react — they may withdraw from their own reaction to someone undergoing such a psychic upheaval (p. 95). Even in a shattered state I found my heart could still break.

I made bad decisions guided by panic about where and how to live. The job I'd taken at the *Virginian-Pilot/Ledger-Star* turned out to be very different from the one I was offered, and in a haze of real-life challenges plus my anomaly career taking off I quit that job and moved into the attic rooms of a friend's mother's house.

In *Healing Shattered Reality* Alice Bryant and Linda Seebach describe a young woman's emotional upheaval after an alien encounter. Her mother and other family members recognize she is in crisis and help her handle the situation accordingly (p. 47). I took pause reading that. How different my anomaly career would have been if I'd been around people with such perception and knowledge.

I think that would be unusual. We humans have a poor record when it comes to handling the extraordinary. In his book *Anatomy of a*

*Phenomenon: Unidentified Objects in Space—A Scientific Appraisal* astrophysicist Jacque Vallee describes how people in Lyon reacted during a time of spaceship sightings. Termed "fiery armies" in Vallee's translated account, these sightings occurred throughout the eastern part of France including Verdun in 972 A.D. In Lyon the archbishop Agobard is "said to have freed several men and a woman who had come down from one of these spaceships" (p. 7). When these "astronauts" later admitted they were "wizards," the villagers mobbed them, rounding them up and killing them, and "their corpses were fastened to boards and thrown into the river" (p. 6-7).

Jacque Vallee also writes in *Anatomy of a Phenomenon* of the profound effect of an encounter with the extraordinary on Ezekiel of biblical fame. After a strange vehicle came down from the sky and landed near the Chebar River in Chaldea (modern-day Iraq) in 593 B.C., Ezekiel was taken aboard then deposited in the Tel Abib Mountains where he "remained 'speechless' for seven days" (p. 2).

## Questioning whether it really happened

My years of living my life in two streams proved to be a boon. Even shattered I could to a degree compartmentalize the experiences and my responses. Not married or partnered, I was on my own, and the wolf was never far from the door. That practical reality plus my own self-doubt about the secret experiences allowed that stream to grow stronger and exist alongside the stream of my anomaly career. I found a temp job working as the front-office admin for a Norfolk engineering firm with government contracts. I'd worked all of my undergraduate years as a part-time Psychology Department secretary at Old Dominion University and had worked on a number of projects funded by the military. At one point during my undergraduate years I started an office services business, and one of my first customers was Allen Ginsberg's editor, Gordon Ball, for whom I transcribed some of Ginsberg's hand-written journals.

I had work now in my nightly dreams: I was assisting the aliens in their physical transition to our planet.

My sister Chrissy and I were both gateways. Gone now were the dreams of the machine-like aliens quietly transmitting their telepathic message to me from across a table. Now they tried to use our voice boxes to vocalize their message that poured down from the sky into us. I don't know what the message was in our words. Physically it looked beautiful as it streamed in silvery, glittery stars into us, doubling us over with its force.

The aliens also needed me as a witness as they transformed themselves from whatever substance or energy they were into beings more like us—air-breathers, speakers of words, emoters. This was their final transformation, and they rolled back the scrim of the sky to show me the universe they had created next to ours. The US military was assisting the aliens but at the same time the aliens protected me from being discovered by the military; I don't know why. I just knew the aliens wanted me as witness to their transformation.

## Physical anomalies

As a teenager and into my early forties I stopped analog watches and clocks. A watch on my wrist would slowly stop keeping time then stop altogether. My dad had the same problem. I had to place alarm clocks across the room so they would reliably go off to wake me up in time. As an adult, it was not unusual for street lights to go out as I passed them, often several in succession. I've heard from others since who have experienced the same phenomenon, so perhaps it is not uncommon.

When the secret experiences shifted out of dream time and began to occur in waking time in the late 1980s, my body began to break down. Red welts appeared like slashes on my back, arms and legs at mysterious provocation. For example, the sun starting to set could set could set off an episode, the red streaks sweeping like flames up and down my body. My feet broke down for unknown reasons, and the only shoes I could comfortably wear were corrective shoes, Red Wing Postman black lace-ups. My uterus began rocking painfully back and forth, like a beaker in a lab being mechanically shaken.

At this time I was frequently losing my place on the time continuum, shifting a bit ahead or behind, my senses registering the sounds and sights of future and past times. If I dropped something, I heard the air waves splitting as the object fell through them with what appeared to be a glacial slowness. What had before only happened in dreams now happened in regular, waking life: people and things appeared as golden columns of shimmering energy; others often could not see me or hear me speak. "The human vessel is broken by the power that rushes through it," writes Monica Furlong in *Visions and Longings: Medieval Women Mystics* (p. 33). Monica Furlong uses the term "transcendent" rather than extraordinary, and sees the power as an independent force. If you are looking for interpretation of or meaning behind the experience, Furlong's take can be a helpful construct. The women Furlong writes of "seem unbearably stressed by the demands of the seismic inner vent, as if it cracks asunder the simple humanness of convention and ordinary awareness and opens into a madness that in turn opens into a different sanity" (p. 33).

While reading Furlong in Minneapolis, where I had moved, I swept my kitchen floor and dreamed of a Jain-like life, every step preceded by the sweep of my broom, gently brushing smaller life-forms out of the way so as not to crush them with my feet. I researched area convents and monasteries where I might spend some time. I found a convent in St. Paul and an order in Minneapolis where for a small fee I cloistered myself for occasional overnight visits.

Despite the exhaustion, red welts, visions and unwanted time-traveling, I had to keep functioning. I had rent and bills to pay. I saw a doctor at the University of Minnesota about the welts and rocking uterus, and all she could say was, "We've never seen anything like it." When I eventually consulted a chiropractor, her diagnosis was burned-out adrenals. She suggested a radical change in my diet, and, with nothing to lose, since by that point the only relief I found was to take the one thing I was allergic to, antihistamines, I followed her suggestion. Within a few months, the turn-around began; the symptoms were relieved. The welts went first, then, within a few years, I was able to wear modest high-heels. I graduated to stilettos at a much later point, in my 40s. My uterus calmed down over a period of several years though once in a while would rock in its mad rhythm up until menopause in my early 50s.

## Emotional pattern development

Looking back I wish I'd had the support and structure in place or within reach to pass more steadily through the effects of the secret experiences. In Virginia in the late 1980s when several profound secret experiences shattered me I fell through the seismic crack into the different sanity Furlong describes. One of my strongest memories is of individuals once close to me withdrawing, and the confusion and pain I felt as a result.

In Dr. Donderi's book mentioned earlier, *UFOs, ETs and Alien Abductions: A Scientist Looks at the Evidence,* he writes of a report conducted on nine individuals who reported alien abduction experiences. They all had in common "anxiety, inner turmoil, weak sense of identity, and suspiciousness of others . . . consistent with the powerlessness and trauma associated with the reported abduction experiences" (p. 132-133). The point of the report, and the study behind it, was not to prove that these individuals had had the reported experiences but instead to find out if individuals reporting such experiences have something mentally or psychologically wrong with them that would cause them to come up with such stories. Interestingly, the psychologist who examined the individuals did not know they had had alien abduction experiences; that was the one detail the individuals were asked not to reveal. After completing her analysis, the examining psychologist Dr. Elizabeth Slater was told all of the nine individuals had reported abduction experiences. In a supplemental report Slater firmly noted the individuals' experiences could not be due to mental disorders (p. 132).

This doesn't prove anyone reporting an abduction experience does not have a mental disorder. However, it helps change a commonly-held belief that all experiencers do. It also helps bolster experiencers' sense of confidence in the truth of what they felt and experienced and, further, treat the results with the gravity they deserve. I felt relief and a sense of a new beginning when I read the details of the Nine Psychologicals report in Donderi's book (p. 132). To begin to believe that what I had experienced was real and that the anxiety and inner turmoil were common to such experiences meant I could envision weaving these things into the fabric of my life.

I didn't have this information in the late 1980s in Virginia. Like the Nine Psychologicals, I certainly was experiencing inner turmoil and a weak sense of self. Those once close to me drew away. The "I" of me was in tatters and my heart was like a wounded animal blindly seeking refuge. "Come home," my parents said, and I did go back, for a time, to those dark, northern woods. I dreamed of knocking, three, loud knocks, and of my entry into witch school. I tried to return to Virginia. I made arrangements, booked a flight and the morning I was to leave I stared out my bedroom window into my parents' backyard and as I envisioned myself returning to Virginia I felt my physical body disappearing. This was terrifying to me. All I could think was "I can't go." I couldn't because I found invisibility too terrifying. Maybe I failed some key test – not ready for enlightenment! Or my humanness won out, as did that of those once close to me in Virginia. I referenced Jean Shinoda Bolen earlier who writes of times when a complex overwhelms the personality and how people around the person may react: they may withdraw, and it may be from their own complex reaction to someone undergoing a psychic drowning. Only in recent years have I

been able to understand and appreciate the fragility of the constellations we move in when in relationship with others.

A few months later, when I'd recovered some sense of self, I moved to Minneapolis, moved into a house I shared with two other women, and found a part-time, temporary job in arts administration at what was then The World Theatre, now The Fitzgerald, where Garrison Keillor's *A Prairie Home Companion* is performed and broadcast. My burning desire to write re-ignited, and I lived a dual life, the two-stream life so familiar to me, rising at 3 am to write and temping in office jobs during the day. My work began to get published. One piece won a fiction award, and in conjunction with that I read the work at a public reading in Duluth, and a short time later was granted a fellowship to a writers' retreat, also in northern Minnesota.

I continued temping. For a while I took the bus to downtown Minneapolis and executed trades for managers of financial portfolios of what was then First Bank. During this period I dreamed the aliens gave me an instrument, a long tube like the Aborigine's didgeridoo. I blew on one end, and tiny white feathers came out the other. This allowed the aliens to metamorphose from their dimension into the physicality of ours.

The morning after this dream, I woke to find tiny white feathers littering the dining room. I was stunned, seeing a remnant from the dream, proof. I stood there, immobilized, unable to process anything. The shock blunted any intelligence I had. Mechanically, I vacuumed the dining room, placed the vacuum cleaner bag in the trash can in the alley.

I took the bus downtown to my temp job. As usual, I walked the skyway to Subway for lunch. I was feeling the fatigue that had begun to plague me and felt rocked by vibrations of those around me as I stood in line for my sandwich. I went back to work, heard my manager walk up behind and begin speaking. When I turned, I saw no one was there. Five minutes later the exact scenario actually occurred, word for word, action for action.

When I returned home from work later that day, I walked out the back door of the house to the alley and put away the empty trash can.

I had a dual career: By day I carried out trades, by night I helped the aliens metamorphose from their dimension into ours.

## Wonder, Extreme Fright, Connection, Adapting

In his article "A Touch of the Witch" Michael Ventura calls people between daily time and the Dreamtime "everyday witches" (p. 5-6). I had chanced upon a clipping of this article on a restaurant bathroom wall in Taos, New Mexico. I read and felt hope and stirrings of belief in what was too new to believe: I was a gateway, and I was not alone.

Perhaps I radiated everyday witchiness early on, a quality that caught beings from other realms. According to my parents when I was as young as three or four I would go off by myself, usually to the bedroom I shared with my older sister, and sit on the floor and be still. At six I stood under a huge pine tree on a mound in the yard of our house in Tacoma, Washington. On overcast fall days I felt something there. That habit was put to good use in later dreams in which I sat quietly in the long, informational sessions with creatures of indeterminate species. I sat passively and quietly across from the being with my eyes open. I didn't try to run away or argue. It was only when I woke that my heart was thudding and my nerves were screaming with red alerts. It seems my lot was tranquility while in the other world, extreme fright once I was back in ours.

Extreme fright is not a good foundation for a stable life in our world as we know it. Nor is splintered consciousness. For me, and for others who've told me their stories, getting our minds blown seems to be a by-product of secret experiences. I've wondered if this could be a directed, intended affect by the intelligence behind secret experiences – what better way to change our humanness than to make us something else from the mental construct up?

Ken Wilber writes in *No Boundaries: Eastern and Western Approaches to Personal Growth* that our belief in ourselves as separate entities is a mental construct that is learned and self-created and that takes one away from "unity of the body and mind, the unity of feeling and attention" or unity consciousness (p. 73). "Unity consciousness is not a particular experience among other experiences, not a big experience opposed to a small experience, not one wave instead of another. Rather, it is every wave of present experience just as it is" (*No Boundary*, p. 127). Could those times when my consciousness dispersed and I no longer held the concept of "me" been times of breaking through to that oneness? Or breaking apart into it.

During this time one of my attempts at reaching out into the world to understand what I was experiencing was to create a course for the University of Minnesota on not just the bizarre but the whole continuum of experiences that pull you out of life. Titled "In the Land Between Heartbeats: Stories of Descent," it offered reading and writing as a way through experiences that pull you out of life. The metaphor of the course relied on the Sumerian goddess Inanna's descent into the underworld, the same employed by Jungian Sylvia Brinton Perera's book on the myth as a psychological metaphor.

The course, offered through the University's Compleat Scholar Program, called men and women who to one degree or another had been expelled from life by an out-of-the-ordinary experience. They, like many of us, did not have the supporting subculture Richard Heckler writes about in *Crossings: Everyday People, Unexpected Events, and Life-Affirming Change* that can offer comfort and guidance when the unexpected shatters you and pulls you out of life:

> If we are surrounded by people who understand the passages
> that we negotiate as we grow—if we are fortunate enough to
> live in a subculture in which tales of the quest, of the hero's
> or heroine's journey, of spiritual transformation are prized
> and told—we may find guidance and inspiration during the
> times we are certain....It doesn't necessarily ensure a safe trip,
> but knowing that our journey has deep historical and spiritual
> roots helps us realize that we are not alone (p. 133).

I expanded my list of experiences the course covered to include the unexpected such as loss, rejection and grief. Those experiences also have the power to knock people out of their orbit and render them stunned.

I assembled a reading list of fiction, poetry and non-fiction that spoke to the experience and could serve as guides. I offered the literary healing of works about the transformative power of deeply-felt experiences, and a forum to talk about these often isolating experiences.

I taught this course for four years, including a brief stint at a center in Winston-Salem, North Carolina. Together with those individuals who the course called, most of them educated professionals, we explored the literary roots of such experiences. We studied examples from literature, and the students performed the writing exercises I developed to accompany the readings and discussions.

For a time each week we had our own subculture. I was gratified for those few hours. I felt relief from the constant weight of shame at what I believed had become a wreck of a life. We all felt shame at our failure and panic as doors closed. "Torschlusspanik" is the German term for that particular panic when you feel the door between you and life's opportunities has closed, writes Heckler in *Crossings* (p.133-134). Further, writes Heckler,

> it connotes the terror of disconnection that ensues when we
> are unable to sense continuity in the unexpected directions
> our lives may take. The source of such powerful anxiety is not

that we have actually become lost, but that we are unable to see these events as part of a larger picture, the picture of ourselves in a passage (p. 134).

Heckler gathered together the stories of several individuals who went through unexpected experiences (as opposed to what I might call extraordinary or anomalous) that jerked them out of life: accidents, hitting a wall due to addictions, the ending of an important relationship, unexplained but pervasive dissatisfaction.

In Heckler's paradigm, these events are on a continuum from slumber to personal evolution. Slumber looks like what most of us would call normal life: routine, home life, day-to-day relationships, work, shopping. In that routine, however, lurk the seeds for disruption. This "Stage of Conventionality," as psychiatrist and author Roger Walsh calls it, by definition must end: waking follows slumber (*Crossings*, p. 132). After periods of feeling lost and rudderless, each of Heckler's percipients eventually came to view their encounters as though they were wake-up calls.

Heckler's interviewees' responses to their experiences seem mostly to occur in the mental realms. Unexpected, out-of-the-ordinary things happened, but nothing that scared the bejesus out of them.

Some of Heckler's experiencers as well as the students in my classes heard voices at various points in their journeys, something I experienced as well. I offered up to my students this statement in Holger Kalweit's work, *Dreamtime and Inner Space: The World of the Shaman*: "Only a few of us who live in modern Western civilization understand that benevolent 'helping spirits' and 'imaginary friends' are by no means projections of an imagination gone riot" (p. vii).

All who took my course, the majority working professionals, had had encounters with the extraordinary and many felt traumatized by these experiences. As I listened to others tell their stories of being shown a new reality and in some cases remade into something different, for the first time I felt a sense of awe. I could be curious about my students' experiences because for once I had company in my anomaly career.

In the mid-1990s, my writing career continued getting some traction. I co-authored a book for teens on understanding the AIDS epidemic. That book and a subsequent book I wrote won awards. I won a travel grant to return to the Dismal Swamp in the southeastern corner of Virginia, and was invited on a trip to Africa along with several others whose work was related to AIDS. At the time I felt I didn't have the money to go on the trip. I can honestly say I didn't, but I wonder why my belief in the plasticity of reality abandoned me at the point. I also began to get some small, freelance writing jobs, one a ghost-writing opportunity for a mental health column, another an article in a local magazine. But even so, I still needed my day jobs to pay the rent and the bills. This reality tempered my ability to feel awe, wonder and curiosity at my secret experiences and those of others I met and got to know through the descent course.

My life began to settle in my late thirties. I had steady employment in technology which meant fewer money worries. I took advantage of a high demand for on-shore technical support help in the early 1990s, before much of that work was moved off-shore. I signed up with another temp agency, took their training to learn how to provide basic computer help desk support, then took my first technical temp job, manning the helpdesk phone, logging incidents for internal corporate customers. Gradually I increased my technical knowledge and abilities and moved into tech support at Dayton's-owned Target in downtown Minneapolis where I helped solve mainframe and network connectivity issues. I took an opportunity to work on a knowledge management project which I leveraged into a permanent position at a local technology company where I combined technical and writing skills in the form of knowledge management.

I dreamed of a little being named something like Beattakukka who sat on the edge of a coffee table in my living room, his legs crossed at the ankle. He was beige all over. This was the only time I dreamed of an extraterrestrial who looked like the type more commonly seen or experienced. "Did all those dreams I had really happen?" I asked him. He smiled and nodded.

I took up yoga at 39, lost 40 pounds I'd gained during my temping years and discovered a stylist who made my hair, naturally the color of nails with white streaks, the perfect shade of champagne. I met Tom, the love of my life, and we married in 2006. When I told him about my secret experiences, characteristically he just listened. I don't know whether he believes these happened or not, but he has always just taken in what I tell him, not offering an opinion either way. He is by nature quiet, patient and reticent, which allowed my feelings to safely flower.

## Shame

Something held me back from talking about my encounters with beings from other planets or dimensions in the University of Minnesota courses I taught. It might have been shame and fear. Most of the people who took my course were educated professionals, and I feared losing their respect. Paulette Salo attributes a fear of people making fun of her to her initial resistance to the mission the angel revealed to her at age 60 while in intensive care (personal communication, January 2014). I also never spoke of my secret experiences during any sort of counseling I undertook over the years. It was not until 2011 when I spoke openly about them. I was between jobs, when my contract job at Best Buy headquarters ended. My hair stylist at the time, Jen, an independent business owner in Savage, Minnesota, introduced me to Bob, a Small Business Development Center adviser who also teaches at Dakota County Technical College. My idea at the time for a small business was a sort of roving writer providing spur-of-the-moment writing help and advice. Throughout my career in office jobs it seemed there was always someone who needed help with a sentence that wasn't quite right, finding the right word, or providing a quick edit of a paragraph. I was usually the person those office people turned to. Why not find a way to make myself available to other office people in need of a quick writing fix? I envisioned a totally mobile service with anonymous service providers all named "Writer Nine."

I planned to offer immediate online assistance at the same time visually marketing the service at lunch time in areas where busy office workers grazed. I would wear a pencil skirt and heels and be furiously at work on my device with discreet signage, "Writer Nine" on a placard next to me. "Yeah, that's just what I need, a writer for that last paragraph of my report," I envisioned a stressed office worker thinking as he waited in the line for his sub and noticed my sign. I'd review and edit in the time it took to get a second sub, and use Square on my device to process credit card transactions.

My husband, my hair stylist and my new small business adviser all agreed I was putting myself at risk for individuals with un-business-like intentions. The fact that didn't occur to me may tell you something about my view of the world or my abilities to sail through it. However, in my initial chat with Bob he mentioned one of his clients based her business on her ability to see angels, and I mentioned my experiences. That blossomed into a full-blown business plan for a service offering including a website, a blog, becoming known as an expert, and eventually a course for other secret experiences along with this book.

I purchased a domain name and started a WordPress blog. I reconnected with hypnotherapist and extraterrestrial abduction researcher Craig Lang, with whom I'd done hypnotherapy in the 1990s. Craig had recently left his full time day job as a software developer to devote himself to his hypnotherapy practice. I told him of my current project, developing a service offering for secret experiencers, and he invited me to tell my story at a MUFON meeting held in New Brighton, Minnesota.

As I told my story, I looked out into an audience whose members' faces were lit with interest and belief. They believed me. They were interested. They were eager to know more. They were also a discerning, critically-thinking audience. When I mentioned my dad's role in running air operations for the Navy on an aircraft carrier off the coast of Vietnam, one of the audience members asked his rank. "Second Lieutenant," I said. Several audience members made scoffing noises, and a general disagreement arose, reminding me of boos and cat-calls that can arise in the broadcast "Prime Minister's Questions." Several of the MUFON audience members seem unconvinced that a man of dad's rank would have been in charge of air operations on an aircraft carrier during Vietnam.

You'd think at this point in my advance through life – I was 52 – I would have had the poise and maturity to calmly address the question. I'd been a speaker at conferences and a lecturer at university; I knew how to speak publicly. I sidestepped the question. Internally I felt sick that somehow I'd gotten a fact wrong. I knew how not to show this but afterwards in reaction to a general sense of shame shut down my efforts to create a service offering around my secret experiences, of which speaking publicly at MUFON was a first step. I tucked away my sheet of hand-written email addresses of interested individuals I'd collected at the MUFON meeting along with my drafts of what you are reading now. I stopped contributing to my secret experiences blog.

I felt the most important thing was finding a job. When an Interactive Producer role came my way in March of 2012 I took it. A part of me knew it wasn't the right fit – basically a project manager for web projects – but I took it anyway. My husband thought it was a good idea, knowing it could lead to a permanent position. I felt carried by his belief in the rightness of taking the job along with the even stronger current of my belief in the redemptive power of work, especially technology-centered work that absorbed me so mentally. Working in technology allowed me to create my own thought-shield, holding at bay anything I didn't want to take a closer look at, with the added bonus of blending in with the general populace.

I did well in the job until organizational changes occurred about a year into the position. For various reasons, I struggled to meet the demands of the job. I'd never struggled to perform at work; this was a new experience for me.

Not excelling at a job was the first step toward cascading realizations: first, that for me work had been a toe-hold to normalcy from an early age. It was a way I could fit in and gain approval from my parents and other important elders. Corporate America loves its hard workers, and I eventually found self-acceptance as one of those workers. However, when my health broke down, so did that construct. As the mental and psychological structure I'd built around me cracked, so too did my outlook. I struggled with depression and crying jags. Eventually with some help I found my way, but not due to self-will. As inner and outer circumstances changed, so passed the belief I must work hard and exhaustively. And as that belief faded, awareness grew of how ashamed I felt for so many years as a result of secret experiences. Craig Lang, who works with experiencers of unusual phenomena, notes we are in relationship with what he calls "visitors," whether we know it or not, and they may be controlling the relationship (personal communication, January 2012). Shame has kept me quiet for many years, even when the public response to my story was for the most part welcoming. If Lang is right, perhaps shame's function is protective. Had I taken my experiences beyond the MUFON audience two years ago, I wouldn't have had the daily-world experiences that broke down my office worker persona and opened up a new way of looking at my secret experiences. The qualities I had been quietly developing blossomed, and here is where the meaning lies.

# 3 MEANING

I believe your best chance at figuring out the meaning behind your secret experiences lies in the process of telling your story. In that telling, you understand what you've become. What new qualities have developed? What latent qualities have come to the fore? How do these qualities affect how you move in the world? During this process read all you can on the topic of anomalous and extraordinary experiences, whether you agree with the views expressed or not. Read the poetry, literature and non-fiction on the transformative aspects of losing yourself, whether to depression, change or extraterrestrial encounter (see the bibliography at the end of this book for some places to start). Let the knowledge sink in while you tell your story. Maybe you will find and connect with others who've had similar experiences; maybe not. Either way, stay close to the literary allies you discover, and the comfort and respite you find in reading their work. This is a strong foundation for the process of telling your story, which in and of itself can lead to inner transformations and an understanding of the meaning of your secret experiences.

This section offers a taste of my process of finding meaning in my secret experiences, describing some of the key pieces of literature that figured in my process, my personal response to them and how they aided in my process.

This section also offers precepts or guidelines to integrating secret experiences. These are based on what worked and what didn't work for me or, should I say, mistakes I made. You can learn from my stumbles.

On that note, here is our first secret experience integration precept: abandon hope of using traditional narrative to tell your story.

Trained as a writer I tried to find meaning in my experiences by putting them in the form of a narrative, a story with a beginning, middle and end. Here is a condensed version of what resulted from taking that approach:

> In the first period of my 30 years of secret experiences, I was introduced to other planets and creatures; in the second, in my teenage years, I sat silently with a solitary alien as it transmitted knowledge into my mind telepathically; in the third, I assisted the extraterrestrials in their transformation to our dimension; and in the fourth, I witnessed their final transformation and the building of the new world beyond ours.

I went in circles with this approach. Edward O. Wilson writes in his book *Letters to a Young Scientist,*

> however much the humanities enrich our lives, however definitely they defend what it means to be human, they also

limit thought to that which is human, and in this one important sense they are trapped within a box. Why else is it so difficult even to imagine the possible nature and content of extraterrestrial intelligence? (p. 170).

Whatever it is you understand about the narrative of your experiences, it is likely it will not lead you to understanding the meaning. Terry Matheson, in his book *Alien Abductions: Creating a Modern Phenomenon* views narrative with suspicion, as though narrative is a construct forced on an experience and designed to influence the reader or listener. He writes, "even the most seemingly insignificant linguistic and rhetorical decisions made in the act of constructing a narrative are determined by those biases of the writer, and cumulatively contribute to how we will respond" (p. 33). I think this is a healthy approach.

Wilson also writes in *Letters to a Young Scientist*, "There is only one way to understand the universe and all within it, however imperfectly, and that is through science" (p. 169). I don't pretend that my methods are scientific; however, it was by going through the process of trial and error to find the shape of story that I came to understand the meaning behind the experiences. The meaning has more to do with what I've become rather than guessing at the extraterrestrials' intent.

If not traditional narrative, then what?

Try my approach: arrange the events of what happened in your secret experiences chronologically but refrain from much scene-setting or description of your emotional state and avoid a narrative arc—avoid rising action, climax or denouement where all the threads are tied together. Box feelings and responses into a separate section and meaning in another. Write, read, reflect; repeat.

Secret experience integration precept: get comfortable with the spiral shape of telling your story, looping through the sections over and over.

The spiral shape, the returning over and over again to the experience, is the one appropriate for ineffable tales of encounters or those that seem beyond words when you are trying to understand their meaning to you.

With each cycle back to the experiences they take on increasingly solid reality. For me, and to my surprise, a feeling of faith in the intelligence behind the experiences began to bud and grow with each pass along the spiral. This faith is in its infancy; who knows what changes are in store for me on the next loop back along the spiral.

I am now winding back to that spot in the spiral where I tell my story, this time better equipped, thanks to Dr. Donderi, and offer this section as a guide to this approach. If you employ it, you may not emerge rich, thin, blonde and beautiful but you will move more confidently through this world and others, perhaps even becoming one who can move and back forth between worlds. Girl in Life Stream One who grew up watching television shows like *Lost in Space*, *Night Gallery*, and *Dark Shadows* envisions doors cut out of air that we humans step through. However, Girl in Life Stream Two knows, at this time, anyway, to get to other worlds we humans fall through cracks we didn't know were there, and those experiences can turn us into different sorts of beings, for example, those who are less visible to those in the world we left behind. I suspect the experience of consciously moving between worlds would be more like Al·lith's in Doris Lessing's' novel, *The Marriages Between Zones Three, Four and Five*, when she leaves the world of solid people and objects for that of the flames. You continue leaving behind who you were to physically become other.

The organization of this section mirrors the path my spiral took, what sources of meaning and interpretation I encountered and digested and how this continued to deepen my understanding. First, we'll look at works that offer a metaphorical explanation for the beings that spirit us away from our world to others where we undergo great change. Second, we'll look at the literature that offers the possibility of these beings being real to the experiencer but ultimately says they are figurative. Third, we'll move to works where the experiencers' stories are conveyed by individuals of academia and science. These writers let the experiencer's nuts-and-bolts stories stand on their own. Some offer judgment or interpretation as to the reality of those experiences and the beings who populate them, some do not. Fourth, we'll move to a work by an individual in science who says extraterrestrial visits are real. Then we'll depart from our study of the subject matter experts who interpret the experiences to those who have the experiences. A view on common new qualities that emerge for experiencers and taking those new qualities into the world is offered in the final chapter.

Worlds of meaning have grown up around narratives of encounters with the extraordinary. The extraterrestrial encounter experience easily lends itself to constructing possible meaning. The reports themselves are often populated with beings, narratives, extraordinary images and sometimes even messages from the other-worldly beings who serve as the guides. Encounters with anomalous beings such as angels and demons have a rich heritage and a ready-made universe of meaning, but even so additional interpretation is always an option. Angel sightings might mean the end of the world is near, or an indication someone has been chosen for something none of us can really explain but clearly it is celestial in nature. Visits from a Man in Black, being rained on by frogs or spontaneously becoming invisible seem the stuff of comic books or a Hollywood script. But if we dig a bit below the American popular culture line, we find serious literary treatment of the effects of encounters with such beings, from experiences from current time to many centuries past.

Those who write about the meaning of encounters with the extraordinary locate the physical reality of the encounters somewhere along a spectrum with "imaginary" on one end, "metaphorical but real psychologically" in the middle, and "actual" on the other end. We'll focus on those works that locate the reality between metaphorical and actual.

In the metaphorical middle of the spectrum, these experiences may be viewed as a vehicle for personal transformation. By "vehicle" I mean the expression or embodiment; the narrative of the experience expresses the tenor of what you recall factually happened.

You might say the encounter with the extraordinary gets you from one spot to another. Once you are in the new spot, the effects of the experience act as a crucible to "melt down" and remake or transform your psyche (switching metaphors here). A crucible is a container that can take temperatures high enough to melt any substance or otherwise alter its content. Likewise, the effects of secret experiences can serve this function for who you are psychologically and in the world. They become a figurative container to melt down who you are in order to change you.

In their book *The Stormy Search for the Self* Christina and Stanislav Grof call experiences of encounters with the extraordinary "spiritual emergencies," "difficult stages of a profound psychological transformation that involves one's entire being" (p. 31). Stanislav Grof, both an M.D. and a Ph.D., is a psychiatrist with over 50 years of experience researching and offering healing for transformative experiences from encounters with the non-ordinary. Perhaps best known for his "holotropic breathwork," Dr. Grof is currently Professor of Psychology at the California Institute of Integral Studies and has served as Chief of Psychiatric Research at the Maryland Psychiatric Research Center and Assistant Professor of Psychiatry at Johns Hopkins University School of Medicine in Baltimore, Maryland.

According to the Grofs spiritual emergencies may

> take the form of nonordinary states of consciousness and
> involve intense emotions, visions and other sensory changes,
> and unusual thoughts, as well various physical manifestations.

These episodes often revolve around spiritual themes…
feelings of oneness with the universe, encounters with various
mythological beings, and other similar motifs (p. 31).

It's interesting to compare these responses to those that
accompany Post-Traumatic Stress Disorder (PTSD) responses, here
from the National Institute of Mental Health (NIMH)
http://www.nimh/nih.gov:

- Re-experiencing the ordeal in memories and nightmares
  or frightening thoughts

- Emotional numbness

- Sleep disturbance

- Depression

- Anxiety

- Irritability or outbursts of anger

- Feelings of intense guilt

- Often try to avoid any reminders or thoughts of the
  ordeal

It was helpful for me to learn that a traumatic experience can
cause you to re-experience the ordeal in thoughts. Whenever I can't
stop the looping tape of thought, I can remember there may have
been a degree of trauma in what I experienced, whatever it might be
(supernatural or not).

Waiting can be a valid response for those who experience any of
the eight secret experiences. Performing simple, homey activities can
also assist the individual experiencing the shock of encounters with
the extraordinary. In the section "Strategies for Everyday Life" in *The*

*Stormy Search for the Self* the Grofs suggest temporarily putting aside more complicated tasks requiring focus and instead taking part in simpler activities such as housecleaning and dish washing. "In many ashrams or monasteries, the same person sweeps the same floor day after day after day," write the Grofs. "This is not just a tedious chore; it is a very straightforward way to balance the tension between worlds" (p. 167).

Sweeping floors was all I wanted to do during some of my most difficult times, when I was slipping in and out of dimensions. However, in my case I swept and worried, anxious about making enough money to pay the rent. Looking back I wish I'd had the presence of mind to notice my desire to just sweep floors during those difficult times. There is respite and comfort in such simple, rhythmic activities.

Secret experience integration precept: heed the call to simple activities.

When you are integrating extraordinary experiences into your normal life you are setting the foundation for all that comes next. This takes enormous energy, physical and psychic. Let your body and conscious mind rest in the comfort of humble activities. You don't have to quit your job as an IT analyst and become a janitor. You can just rest in the comfort of sweeping the floor. If your mind jumps to worries, you might use Buddhist nun Pema Chodron's (and other Buddhists') suggestion to simply label those thoughts, "thinking." This keeps the thoughts light as air, letting them float out of your mind. When they float back in, again label them, "thinking." I am only touching on meditation here, not intending to offer a full discourse on its benefits.

Refrain from doing what I did. I was so worried about money I missed the possible opportunity that sweeping my kitchen, a quiet, rhythmic activity, would have begun weaving my two life streams together. I try not to torture myself too much with thoughts of missed opportunities, and console myself with the notion that my path is what it is. But you can learn from my mistakes and benefit from what I discovered.

Just as meaning of secret experiences occurs on a spectrum so too do secret experiences. On one end they may cause mild depression; on the other they may pull you out of life and shatter you. Whoever you were, you no longer are. Wherever you were, you no longer are. And yet you cannot move forward. Not where you used to be, but not yet where you're going, you may feel stuck, abandoned, lost.

Psychologically you've descended, like Sumerian goddess Inanna whose underworld sister hung her on a peg where she turned to rotting meat. Inanna may be new to you. In our culture our knowledge of gods and goddesses is mostly based on those in the Greek and Roman pantheon. Zeus, for example, the ruler of Mount Olympus, is familiar to most of us. He stands at the ultimate strategist and finds his contemporary counterpart in a powerful, successful CEO. Athena, the daughter Zeus bore from his head, may also be a familiar Greek goddess. Like her father, she is a strategist, and finds her parallel in a successful, corporate businesswoman. Persephone, the eternal girl, and Apollo, the boy wonder, are also

Greek figures you may be familiar with. Inanna's story, also known as the Babylonian Isthtar's descent, takes place in Uruk, modern-day Iraq, and is one of the oldest recorded stories yet it was only discovered and translated in the last century.

In Inanna's descent story I found the mirror I was so hungry for, a story where the heroine is reduced to nothing yet ultimately emerges from the underworld with new qualities (though some of those new qualities do not work out so well for those on the receiving end when Inanna returns above-world). I read Diane Wolkstein and Noah Kramer's translation but stayed closest to Sylvia Brinton Perera's work, *Descent to the Goddess: A Way of Initiation for Women*. A Jungian psychotherapist, Perera describes the experiences of a descent as "sacred process" and offers the myth as a metaphor for contemporary women's experience of a psychological descent (p. 58). Full disclosure: her book gave me hope that there was meaning to my experiences. While I clung to T.S. Eliot's poetic suggestion to "wait without hope" as though to a lifeline in truth I was desperate for hope. Eliot, born in the US and eventually a British subject, wrote this phrase in his poem "East Coker," part of a larger work, *Four Quartets,* published in 1943.

Secret experience integration precept: let hope live in your heart but don't make specific plans based on it.

Looking back, I would say I might have moved faster and more easily into my new reality had my hopes reflected a general optimism or faith instead of specific, concrete hopeful plans. I probably short-circuited a general direction or path in my development. It's easy to be smart in retrospect.

Let hope live in your heart but let it be hope that everything will be alright, because it probably will, but perhaps not according to your plan or goals. This is time to let go of what Sylvia Brinton Perera refers to as "goal-directed development," a way of approaching life that has caused us to lose familiarity with the natural ebb and flow of life or, as Perera writes in *Descent to the Goddess* "unity with nature and the cosmos" (p. 14). In other words, this is not the time to make plans. From my own experience, I would caution against hoping for any specific outcome. Hold that for later once you've returned to the surface. When you have been changed by secret experiences, it is unlikely you can ever go back to where you were or who you were. It's natural to hope to return to the comforts of your previously-known life. You probably won't be able to. Maybe in form but not likely in practice or spirit. The key is finding a way to keep your mind on its new track. When it goes back to its old track, and it probably will, you will find yourself making plans and strategies based on that old life. And there you will probably run into resistance that will deplete your energy and break your heart.

Assume you will be crazed with hope to get back to "normal." When your heart is broken and your mind is blown, when you're invisible to people in your own dimension, and your new job is helping extraterrestrials evolve on your planet, it's difficult not to feel crazed with hope that you will get out of the situation and get back to what you once knew as normal. Assume this won't happen.

Jacqueline Winspear writes in her novel *Leaving Everything Most Loved*, "Leaving that which you love breaks your heart open. But you will find a jewel inside, and this precious jewel is the opening of your heart to all that is new and all that is different, and it will be the making of you—if you allow it to be" (p. 236).

Perera refers to the "one cosmic power" encountered in descents, a "living balance" that is possible only after our ego, that part of ourselves that moves about in the world and gets things done, is shaken to the core (p. 14). Perhaps in earlier, nature-focused cultures our egos didn't need so much shaking. Perhaps then we were more aligned with natural rhythms related to crops and the stars. By this I mean the natural ebb and flow of life as opposed to aiming for constant or continuous improvement to ourselves, our relationships and our work. Inanna equates to our Venus, a planet that is visible in either the morning or evening sky then for a time appears to disappear before again returning to visibility.

"Our planet is passing through a phase," Perera writes, "the return of the goddess—presaged at the beginning of the patriarchy in this myth [Inanna's]" (p. 15). And so we are linked to our own planet's phases which in turn are likely linked to others'.

Similar to the Grofs, Perera recommends waiting as the only antidote to such a process. Waiting may be difficult without allies, and it may be a time when you have few of those. Literature and writing were my allies during the most difficult times, when I felt shattered by encounters with the extraordinary and lost my way –

friends turned away, jobs didn't work out and everything I knew myself to be, my identity, how I moved in the world, was gone.

When I turned to the literature I loved, it provided an abundant return of its own, offering solace and leading me to other, related works. The words from Eliot's "East Coker" became my polestar during this time:

> I said to my soul, be still, and wait without hope
>
> For hope would be hope for the wrong thing; wait without love,
>
> For love would be love of the wrong thing; there is yet faith
>
> But the faith and the love and the hope are all in the waiting.
>
> Wait without thought, for you are not ready for thought:
>
> So the darkness shall be the light, and the stillness the dancing (*Four Quartets*, p. 28).

To wait without hope, to not have a plan goes against almost all the ways our American culture has taught us to deal with adversity. I'm not disparaging that teaching; I'm as much a product of it as anyone. However, it was of no use when I experienced the profound changes as a result of secret experiences. I'd had little preparation for waiting.

Angel artist Paulette Salo notes,

> The angels prepare you in all kinds of ways. The hardest part for most people is the wait....I do think they [the angels] have a master plan, and the person is the one who sets the timeline. It took time for me to get my life in a place where I could actually do it. I was thinking about it a lot and

wondering so that's part of it too. I just had grown at that point [when I could accept my mission]; I'd had enough experiences, and I was just ready (personal communication, January 2014).

As mentioned earlier, on one of the nights before the dream in August 1987 that was the final shattering of me, I dreamed I passed through seven gates in darkness. By the time I was developing the course I had discovered my dream had mythological parallels: Inanna of Sumer descends through seven gates to pay respects to her newly-widowed sister, and an article of clothing is removed at each one until she arrives naked in the underworld (the original strip-tease, as Perera notes).

In the descent course the reading selections and writing exercises mirrored the seven gates in my dream. Each week my students and I went through a gate. The classroom experience was designed to function as a container for the unbearable feelings that often accompany the conscious recollection of experiences that take you out of life. The overall course experience was designed as literary therapy to help those participating understand their traumatic experience and how to move forward.

Most of my students had, like me, fallen through a crack in consciousness as a result of either secret experiences or quieter experiences like those Richard Heckler describes in his work, *Crossings: Everyday People, Unexpected Events, and Life-Affirming Change*. Heckler is a psychotherapist who works with people who undergo life-altering experiences often of a nature not always of this world. He notes in the prologue that in his work he discovered that "there exists levels of information and guidance that lay beneath consensual reality" (p. xvi). His book offers the stories of those individuals he worked with and how their experiences intersected with the extraordinary or, more often, the unexpected. These encounters can lead down a path with distinct phases Heckler identifies: the Slumber, the Call, the Incubation, the Search for Meaning, the Leap and the Integration.

For those in Heckler's stories and for my students and me, the fall through a crack in consciousness shattered old ways of life and in many cases introduced us to new modes of consciousness. Almost none of us sought these out. Almost all longed to return to their former sense of home, the one thing none of us could do.

If you prefer contemporary descent stories and themes, here are some options: for stories of those who descend, watch Mel Gibson's fictional character Max in the original movie *Mad Max* or read the story of Margaret Atwood's main character in her novel, *Surfacing*; for an exploration of the fruits of being on the border between two figurative states read *LaFrontera / Borderlands* by Gloria Anzaldua; for instruction on consequences of not inviting cast-off parts of yourself to the party, try the fairy tale *Sleeping Beauty*. To return to a Greek goddess, consider another look at a lesser-known goddess, Hecate, goddess of the crossroads. Her story and its intersection with Demeter, goddess of the harvest who Hecate accompanies during her time of grieving and wandering, can serve as a guide when you aren't where you used to be but aren't yet where you're going.

Perhaps one day there will be an agreed-upon list of common qualities that humans develop after secret experiences. For now, I can offer a reporting of what I've heard people say happens for them, a list arrived at anecdotally rather than scientifically. I gathered the following list of emotional and physical changes in individuals after prolonged / multiple secret experiences while teaching the descent course from 1994 to 1998 when I met others undergoing transformation and spent several, rich years immersed in the language and literature of evolving inner worlds. My students had experienced contact with the extraordinary or anomalous worlds and creatures. Most of these adult learners were gainfully employed as professionals in their fields and sought community for their secret experiences which the course offered. My own changes are included with theirs:

- Perceptual changes; for example, seeing people as columns of light and a more acute sense of vibrational level of reality

- Shifting back and forth on time continuum (perceived through senses)

- Physical changes; for example, changes in body shape and sharper hearing and sense of smell

- Increased psychic abilities

- Increased intuition manifesting in bodily symptoms; e.g., break-through bleeding day before 9/11

- Preference for silence and low lights (need for reduced sensory stimulation).

Some of Heckler's experiencers as well as the students in my classes heard voices at various points in their journeys, something I experienced as well. I offered up to my students Holger Kalweit's work, *Dreamtime and Inner Space: The World of the Shaman*, referenced earlier, and we all found comfort to in his message that it is our modern Western civilization that is suspicious of friendly spirits whispering help to us. Kalweit's work was as close as I got to offering literature that said the beings that populate anomalous experiences are nuts-and-bolts real. His work felt safe, focusing as it does on shamans. Kalweit, a German ethnologist and psychologist, has studied shamanism in Hawaii, the American Southwest, Mexico, and Tibet, according to his biography on Shambhala Publications (http://www.shambhala.com/authors/g-n/holger-kalweit.html)

Shamans' reality might include actual beings from other times and dimensions. That was palatable. But the average person having the same experiences and calling them real? This seemed to edge into territory neither I nor my students were ready to venture into.

Tellingly, I didn't include John Mack's works in the course.

John E. Mack was a Harvard Medical School professor of psychiatry and Pulitzer Prize-winning biographer. He worked with individuals who reported "alien encounter" experiences.

The John E. Mack Institute web site offers several transcriptions of talks by experiencers (http://johnemackinstitute.org/). These offer some tantalizing theories about meaning. In one the narrator notes, "And I feel that the reason why they [aliens] are not directly with us right now, why they're not walking through the hall right now is because they recognize that it's very difficult for us to get together. I don't know why. But they're posing a problem, and the problem is that they want to coexist with us, but the question is how do we do that? I don't know the answer to that but it's something that we should work on. And I feel it's very important" (http://johnemackinstitute.org/2000/10/ ) .

I resisted embracing such interpretations. I was skeptical of reports that gave human qualities to the visitors' thinking. In the example above the visitors a) recognize it's difficult for humans and extraterrestrials to get together and b) are posing a problem which is they want to coexist with us but question how to do that. They have these pedestrian thoughts but feel they are too different from us to get together? I was resistant as well because I lacked an ability to fully imagine the content of these kinds of reports, to give the presented reality a life in my mind. In my own experiences I had never come away with such certainty about what "they" were about, and I couldn't get comfortable embracing these messages some experiencers brought back. To me they seemed like conjecture. I was still trying to use the rules of our waking world to prove them.

I embraced the descent approach when I feared ridicule if I spoke of things and beings I encountered as real entities. My parents, who were co-experiencers of one of my secret experiences and who had at least one of their own, asked me not to write about the experiences. I think they feared the same ridicule I did or embarrassment. My mother often spoke of her father whose clairvoyance was a source of fear and shame for him, something spoken of in hushed tones

69

between him and her mother, yet, ironically, stunning to the family when the clairvoyance occurred. It certainly wasn't as though he could hide what he saw, his Kansas City, Missouri, music store burning down; he saw it in a dream and promptly called the fire department. The store was, in fact, burning in real life as it burned in his dream. My grandfather also saw his son gunned down in World War II and indicated no surprise when the telegram came.

There's what happens to us, and then there's what we think about what happens to us, an astrologer in Alabama once said to me. Now that my parents have passed on and it's been a long time since I called my job a "career," I feel freer to speak of the reality of the beings I encountered and what I experienced. I may or may not be able to solve their mystery. I think of the ancient Eleusinian Mystery rituals and the secrecy surrounding them. Not knowing and not saying is okay. The process still occurs. Angel artist Paulette Salo echoes this:

> Had the angels told me what my mission was in my first or second near-death experience at 20 and 33 I couldn't have done it. I had kids to get through college. It wasn't until the last one left and my mother passed that I was free to do this work. It takes so much time. It was a journey just getting here (personal communication, January 2014).

"An invisible phenomenon is always stalking us and manipulating our beliefs. We see only what it chooses to let us see, and we usually react in exactly the way it might expect us to react," writes John Keel of *Mothman Prophecies* fame (*The Complete Guide to Mysterious Beings*, p. 319).

As noted earlier hypnotherapist and anomaly researcher Craig Lang, who works with experiencers of unusual phenomena, says we are in relationship with what he calls "visitors," whether we know it or not, and they may be controlling the relationship.

Lang offers the observation that there are two levels of secret experiences.

> One level is the experiences that the experiencer doesn't feel they can share with other people.... That's probably the most difficult aspect of being an experiencer. Then there are the secrets that the phenomenon keeps from you, the experiencer. This is the sense of mystery, the puzzlement, the underlying fear of the unknown that is so pervasive in the life of the experiencer. This is one time when hypnotherapy can be a truly invaluable help—coming to terms with the experience, better understanding of what is going on in the hidden side of life. It's what David Jacobs called the "Secret Life" of the experiencer (personal communication, January 2012).

In his book *The Cosmic Bridge* Lang takes a scientific approach to discerning the nature of the visitors, bridging the details of the experiencers' stories to arrive at contact models to answer the question, "Why are the visitors here?"

He reviews what appear to be extraterrestrials' or ETs' strategies to close or bridge the cosmic gap between ETs and humans. The strategies are based on the reports from those who experience contact with the visitors, both those Lang has worked with individually and those whose experiences are documented by others. Some of the more common reports involve the seeming lack of human choice in the visitor experience, leading to the hypothesis that ETs are hostile and intent on taking over our planet; unexplained pregnancies during which the fetus disappears, leading to the hypothesis that ETs' contact strategy involves genetics and reproduction; a dearth of physical evidence from ETs' visits, leading to the hypothesis the visits must be covert and the ETs' presence kept hidden so they may safely observe us in what to them is a managed preserve (and what to us is our world where we roam unfettered and ignorant); reports of experiencers being shown cataclysmic views of our planet and solar system, leading to the hypothesis a kindly, more superior race is attempting to educate us while there is still time; experiencers reporting developing new psychic skills and experiencing expanding consciousness as a result of visitor contact, leading to the hypothesis that ETs wish to assist us in our psychic development and become better cosmic citizens.

Lang arrives at a combined hypothesis and suggests the ETs visit to "alter humanity," facilitate our evolution so we might grow beyond our current state of consciousness and join the "cosmic community" (*The Cosmic Bridge*, p. 164-167).

Lang is analytical and scientific by trade; he spent many years in computer science and applies the same careful logic and thought to laying out and examining the ET visitor experience, including postulating about ET motivations based on the effects on the experiencers or what they become.

Taking a similar scientific approach but arriving at a different conclusion, Dr. Don Donderi lays out the facts and scientific analysis from his vantage point of a trained professional in the area of human senses. In his book *UFOs, ETs and Alien Abductions: A Scientist Looks at the Evidence*, he opens with three particular close encounters, noting that they describe "something new in the world that I helped to report. These cases begin to explain why UFOs are real and why they are extraterrestrial; the rest of the book continues the story" (p. xi).

"UFOs are real." Reading those words and that introduction and then the rest of the book changed everything for me, as I have mentioned before. I needed a scientist to publicly say UFOs are real before I could believe it myself, in spite of my experiences. In turn I couldn't give my secret experiences or myself as experiencer enough credence to be my starting point for understanding. I relied on the subject matter experts, all of whom stopped short of saying these experiences were nuts-and-bolts real. I adopted that stance as well. I had no idea that thinking kept me from fully understanding and processing the experiences. When my thinking changed after reading Donderi's book, clarity came quickly. I stopped asking "Was it real?" and "What are they?" and instead asked "What am I after years of encounters?" The answer to that question can begin to explain the intelligence that is behind the encounters. As someone with 30-plus years of secret experiences who hid that life, I highly recommend starting with Donderi's book. He shows the way to change your thinking.

There was a waterfall effect by reading Donderi's book and my beliefs shifting to include the reality of my secret experiences. One of these effects was to feel a strong heart-belief and faith in the sentient beings behind my experiences. I've always struggled with faith in any god, Christian or otherwise, though I've been able to embrace something with greater power than mine. Finally following Craig Lang's suggestion, I've begun developing a relationship with these beings based on this blossoming feeling of faith in them in my heart. This could be an imaginary, one-sided relationship; there is no way to know. But isn't that the nature of faith?

# 4 TAKING NEW QUALITIES INTO THE WORLD

In my early 40s my secret experiences began to taper off, and I thought I had reached the end of my anomaly career. I began sleeping through the night. I gained half an inch in height.

Then on September 10, 2001, I had break-through bleeding, something I'd never had before. About 12 hours later, al-Qaeda terrorists attacked the United States, crashing two hijacked commercial airplanes into the World Trade Center twin towers in New York City and another into the Pentagon in Washington, D.C. The fourth crashed into a field in Pennsylvania after the passengers tried to overcome the hijackers. Close to three thousand individuals died in the attacks.

I compared notes with a friend of mine who was strongly intuitive. About 10 years younger than me, she too had experienced break-through the day before 9/11. I considered her intuitive life stream to flow more naturally alongside her daily-world life stream than was the case for me, and this was the first time our bodies had synced up with what appeared to be early warnings.

I began listening more closely to my body in case any other messages came through. I performed informal experiments, observed and recorded what was happening to me physically then scanned global news to determine if my body continued to alert me. I focused on large-scale disasters. Immediately after 9/11 the news stayed focused on that event, so the only big disasters reported, it seemed, were those caused by weather. I have never been prescient about the weather, and my body bore that out by not reacting to impending tsunamis.

However, during this exercise I found my body's sweet spot is catching people with mean-hearted intent (not helpful if that person is your boss). When I sense that intent I am not unlike the proverbial canary in the coal mine: I am overcome, and I fall from my perch. I am not like Deanna Troy, the fictional Star Trek empath who processes intuitive input like a computer processing data. When someone's intent is to do something that will cause loss or harm to others, it emanates like an invisible cloud from them, enveloping me, and all I can think is, "Something bad's going to happen." That's about as smart as I get. I never seem to get any better at managing such situations in the workplace, and I have always been right about sensing what's to come. This is not a great combination. I am like a demoted version of Cassandra of Greek lore: not only does no one believe me, but I can't even articulate what's coming. I can only shake in my boots. In the last few years I have gotten smart enough to not say anything about what I'm feeling to co-workers or friends. I only tell my husband, and rely on him to be the litmus test: given what I'm sensing and what's actually occurring, what do you think is happening?

If this is a solitary time for you and there is no one to ask, oracles can be good sounding boards. One type of oracle, the I Ching, measures the moment, to paraphrase C.J. Jung, Swiss psychologist. The easiest oracle to consult is the tarot. Think of the situation while holding any tarot deck in your hands. Ask, "What's going on in this situation? What am I not seeing?" Then shuffle the cards, cut the deck and turn the top card face up. Turn one more face up and place it cross-wise on top of the first. The first card represents the nature of the situation, the second what is crossing you. For me the crossing card almost always represents what I'm missing. Like Hephaestus, the only working god among the other Greek gods, I can get lost in my subjective feelings and lose my ability to see objectively when my intuition is overwhelmed. This may not be the case for you, and instead the card crossing might mean what's the challenge for you in the situation or what's feeling like conflict.

"Watch what happens." This is also good advice. It comes from Stephanie, an Iyengar yoga teacher in a workshop she led at the St. Paul Yoga Center in St. Paul, Minnesota. It also comes from Michael Ventura in his essay "A Touch of the Witch" and, in a slightly different form, from the poet T. S. Eliot in his poem "East Coker" In *Four Quartets.*

A few years ago I learned how to administer Reiki, a Japanese form of relaxation (and some say healing) at Level II certification. When I give Reiki to humans, critters or non-sentient things, images and pictures float up in my mind but I don't verbalize them (unless the receiver is human and has asked me to) and I try not to attach any meaning to them. To me it feels aggressive to let them harden into a story and force that story on the Reiki receiver. I watch the images come up, I watch them go down.

You can practice watching what happens starting now. You need not believe in what you see and perceive to do this. It may be whatever's behind the experiences already believes in you. "Does it believe in us, that's the question," writes Barbara Kingsolver in her novel *The Poisonwood Bible*. The narrator notes her family's lack of intellectual belief in voodoo spirits but acknowledges

> there was some dark thing out there watching us from the
> forest and coiling under people's beds at night, whether you
> call it fear or the dreaming of snakes or false idolatry or
> what—it's still something. It doesn't care what prayers we say
> at bedtime, or whether we admit we believe in it (p. 428).

However, the degree to which you take your new qualities into the waking world does depend on the degree to which you believe in the reality of the force behind the experiences. Like the Congolese boy in Kingsolver's novel, you may beg to be taken in by those close to you, fully believing in the thing's reality. Or, like me, you may separate your secret experiences into their own life stream and view the force behind the them as real but metaphorical. Nothing bad need come from this, other than that aching sense of a hidden life not fully lived.

Process is also key—most of the steps can be taken in any order: create a factual accounting of your secret experiences; read our existing stories of transformative experiences; take the time to discover and articulate new qualities; maybe find others like you. I think it is helpful to do this step first, if you can: find a way to believe in the reality of the secret experiences. I hope this book offers help in taking all these steps.

I would be interested to hear from secret experiencers how they fare when trying to consciously enter the other worlds they've been introduced to. I have tried this, and haven't been successful, though in truth I'm not sure what success in these worlds would look like.

As I've previously mentioned, I recently met angel artist Paulette Salo. For her, consciously entering the world she'd been introduced to meant accepting her mission. When she did, at about age 60, "The angels brought many opportunities to me; doors just opened" (personal communication, January 2014).

For a time in 2012, when I was between jobs and had started a blog, I consciously set about willing an increase in time in other-worldly realms.

What if I could shift that ratio and choose to spend more time in that other realm? What if when the waking world calls I just turn away? What if through the quality of my attention I shift meaning from what we call this waking life to that other life in which I've been visited by other-worldly beings?

As a result of this willful attempt, I had several interesting dreams about family and blogged about one of my brother in an entry titled "The Dream of Waking Life." In my new, real world, my brother was part cat. I told him I knew our dad's spirit was still with us. He mostly ignored me, as he does in regular, waking life. However, as he curled around his water dish he told me sneaks into our dead dad's house each night and pretends he lives there (view the blog at http://secretexperiences.wordpress.com/2012/02/05/the-dream-of-waking-life/).

And then what happened? I got a job offer as a contract Interactive Producer at a company in downtown Minneapolis in March 2012, working through a staffing firm for creative positions. Like Hephaestus at his forge, I went to work, slipped back into that rhythm I know so well, and that rhythm became what I aligned my life to. I let the Secret Experiences blog go though I sporadically continued working on the book.

The company offered me a permanent position in December 2012. Just a few months later the company reorganized my area, and by spring of 2013 I felt the familiar inner foreboding. Inwardly I felt sick and distraught most of the time, fighting off the feelings of dread threatening to overwhelm me. I searched for another position. I prayed, something I had only recently begun doing with real feeling. My prayers were simple, asking for a calm mind for whatever was coming next. My daydreams on the commuter bus home focused on natural disaster removing the change agents from my workplace (for example, a flood that wouldn't kill anyone but would disrupt operations for weeks). I just wanted whatever was happening to stop so the assault on my inner state would stop, and my inner point-man could stop nervously pacing the battlements.

In the midst of all this I had simple clairvoyant dreams, for example a very vivid dream that one of our executive leaders was writing a book about his business experiences. When I mentioned this to his assistant she confirmed in fact he was.

Then the call came at the end of October. My position along with several others was being eliminated due to changes at the company. All I could feel was relief. A freelance editing job came my way with work for November, and I had a small severance. I resumed work on this book and the accompanying service offering.

So once again I'm getting a break from the iron forge. Without my daily office job, I find I get a solid, almost visceral sense of certain key things about people. Here are two examples: First, in a restorative-style yoga class I attended recently at Yoga 4 You the teacher positioned her mat so it was a hub and the students' mats the spokes. We sat in our wheel-shape in the darkened room, and the teacher, Elle, began speaking. She faced my part of the room. I sat on a mat just to her right. As she spoke, I felt her yoga-teacher persona and her private self viscerally, as though they were two solid things. Second, at the same yoga studio on another visit, I glanced out the door as I pulled off my boots and my eye was caught by a gentleman coming to the door. I got a wave of that combination knowledge and feeling and could feel his sense of agency about the studio. When he entered he didn't immediately approach the front desk but stood slightly back again with that strong sense of agency. He exchanged a look with Kelly, one of the owners, and I knew he must be her husband, which it turned out he was. Like Clever Hans the horse that could do arithmetic, was I just perhaps keenly watching these people around me for physical clues about who they were in the world? Well, that's not a bad way to move. Imagine taking in all that information about a person and carefully weighing it before acting or speaking.

This is one of the ways secret experiences have changed me. For me this particular new way of moving in the world provides meaning to my experiences and also tells me something about the intelligence behind them and how they move in their world and ours.

Secret experience integration precept: The key to finding meaning in secret experiences to take into the world is going through the process of coming to understand them. Your heart and mind must find their way together through understanding, and the meaning will slowly crystallize.

I believe this is so because of our current lack of supporting images of secret experiences in our waking world.

Jean Shinoda Bolen writes in her book *Goddesses in Older Women* of the experience of dreaming of an image then seeking it out in waking life to understand its meaning (p. xxvi). There is a synchronicity between the images people encounter in their dreams and then in real life when undergoing psychological change. The pattern of the archetype shows itself, a forerunner to that development in the person. People who have this experience may feel supported by the synchronous appearance of the images. For example, Bolen writes of women who identify with particular goddesses then discover their symbols have been populating their dreams or walls of their home for some time (p. xx).

People undergoing secret experiences may not experience this synchronicity. For those who have an anomaly career, the images we encounter and take with us are rarely seen in waking life; the images of our transformation rarely make it to the light of day where we spend the majority of our time. Quoting Budd Hopkins, Craig Lang notes that 99.9% to .01% is the ratio of time experiencers spend in the waking versus night-time world where encounters with unusual phenomena often take place (personal communication, April 2014).

When we try to bring our new reality to into this one and tell others we often encounter disbelief and, not surprisingly, no welcoming mirror of the images that haunt us. It seems secret experiences haven't yet fully flowered in our culture into archetypes.

Paulette Salo is assisting in that flowering. She's created over 10,000 images of angels as part of her mission to get people to talk to their angels. She began by painting the guardian angels of terminally ill children who could already see their own angels and would correct details as Salo rendered them (personal communication, 2014).

Ten years after my secret experiences have calmed down, I can now say to myself, these things happened. They had a profound impact on my life. I now assume the truth of what I experienced and felt afterwards. The burning bush may or may not be God, but if you get close enough to get burned, you are stuck with dealing with the physicality of the encounter.

In what ways did the burning bush burn my hand or mark me or change how I operate in the waking world? Here are a few:

I seem naturally to have lucid dreams. Lucid dreams are those dreams in which you become aware you are dreaming. I don't employ techniques to encourage myself to wake up in dreams; I just do. It happens randomly. Besides the lucid dream of my father after he passed, another earlier example is from May 2010 when I woke up inside my dream to a demon burrowing against my chest for warmth. Here is that entry from my journal:

> 5/29/10 – A demon sitting on my chest woke me up. His limbs and torso were long and lanky, though he was miniature, like a large cat. His skin was scaly and he was hairless. His eyes were large, peering out from his bony, old-man head. I had caught him trying to burrow against my chest for warmth. It was his heaviness that woke me. I'm not sure if I saw him with second sight behind closed lids or with regular sight, eyes open. Startled, he met my gaze and with a look of non-reaction faded into transparency as a result.

My sense of smell and touch is sharpened.

My intuition is as much a sense for me as any of the five other.

That same hyper-aware sense of vibrations that blossomed into existence in August 1987 has never left me. I'm not sure if it's intuition or a new ability. It doesn't feel like a gut feeling, but maybe gut feelings are its grosser manifestation. Sensing vibrations doesn't feel surprising any more when it happens; after all, it's been happening for 25 years. As an example of how this manifests, if I am lying awake in the morning in bed with my husband, I can feel his physical stirrings before they become physical. At this point there is no movement; he is still deeply asleep. It's as though I can sharply feel intent. In this example, within a few minutes of feeling the vibration of his intent to move, he shifts a bit on his back and starts the slow process of waking. Another example is on a multi-lane highway. Without stopping to think about it, I can sense when a driver in a certain car is going to put their blinker on and cross over into my lane. It doesn't seem like anything extraordinary to sense this; the same way I take for granted that I hear sounds and see things throughout my waking hours I also take for granted the sensing of vibrations or intent.

I spend less time doing and more time watching and waiting, borrowing from Michael Ventura's advice for what he calls "everyday witches," people between daily time and the Dreamtime, in his article, "A Touch of the Witch" (p. 5-6). How do they handle encounters with the extraordinary? Ventura writes, "They wait and see, take in the information, wait to know what to do with it, proceeding gently—sensing that gentleness is the only antidote, in these realms, to mistakes and fear" (p. 6).

After my trouble with physical invisibility in the late 1980s and early 1990s I am once again finding, as 2013 draws to a close, people are not fully registering my physical presence. I don't know if this means I am actually experiencing physical invisibility again. For example, in the yoga studio I mentioned earlier I greeted a fellow yoga practitioner who I'll call Jack, and he didn't respond back though looked in my direction. He left the lobby to place his mat in the studio, and when he returned he again looked in my direction and said, "Oh, I didn't realize you were here." Another fellow yogi, Lisa, kept physically running into me when she first started attending classes at this same yoga studio. Later when we had gotten to know each other she said she just didn't see me. Hard to scientifically prove anything about these situations, but the elements are similar to when I have experienced spontaneous invisibility to multiple people.

If spontaneous invisibility is what happens by willfully seeking out other realms, I'm ready for it this time and willing to continue this exploration. Yoga serves as a vehicle for this. During a home yoga practice I used a breathing technique I learned in a Yin yoga practice, and for a second my body disappeared. This was not expected or my intent; it was serendipitous. Here's that entry from my journal:

> 12/23/09 – I've been practicing a certain breath in my yoga
> practice learned in a yin yoga practice several months ago—
> thinking of all things coming together on the inhale, action on
> the exhale. At the same time I've been playing with the
> notion that my consciousness can leave my body and perhaps
> go other places. I've tried sending it out in crow pose, since I
> feel the most able to take a high, detached view of things in
> that pose. This a.m. in Sirsasana I practiced the yin breath and
> for a second my body disappeared, or I felt it to be so. Aha!
> That's it. The breath doesn't go anywhere, but the body
> leaves the breath. A bit like death.

I hear what is not spoken or is below the hearing range of regular humans (woof!). For example, when I took Reiki training from David in Lakeville, Minnesota, as I stood off to the side and just behind David I heard a mumbling behind him. I couldn't quite make out the words, but could hear words being spoken though they were too slurred for me to make out what they were. When I mentioned this later to David he smiled and said his guide speaks to him on that particular side. If I couldn't make out the specific words, he said, I wasn't meant to. Of course, this is the kind of logic that makes me nutty. How can you argue with such circular reasoning, asks Girl in Life Stream One? Girl in Life Stream Two doesn't argue and just takes in the fact she heard a teacher's invisible guide mumbling instructions to him.

One night I dreamed my sweet companion Margaret the cat was waiting for me outside the gates of heaven into which she'd woven my name in lights. I woke and felt dread; I knew this wasn't a happy dream. I stumbled about in the darkened house until I found her dying under a low table, gasping for breath as her heart failed and stopped a few minutes later.

A few months before we knew my mom had anything wrong with her, I dreamed she took me into an empty theater and said, "Let me tell you about death." Shortly after she was diagnosed with cancer. As she was undergoing chemotherapy, my appetite matched itself to hers, waning at the same times hers did (we were several hundred miles apart and only compared notes later). My lack of appetite told me where she was in the chemotherapy cycle. About a month before she died I dreamed of the word "Mother" appearing in lights across the night sky. (This dream usually spooks most folks. "Don't dream of my name in lights," they say, as though my dreaming powers the event.)

## Girl One and Girl Two Integrate

I woke up at 2:16 am on Wednesday, December 18, the day before my 55th birthday, and felt my previously hidden side flowering. Girl in Life Stream Two was rising to my psychological surface like cream rising to the top. I lay there in the dark, my husband asleep beside me, and felt myself to be fully who I am, as though for years I'd been hiding a mermaid's tail and finally dropped the costume. I felt an expansive sense of self and peace. I haven't felt that often during my years of Girl in Life Stream One being at the helm. She was busy for many years making her way in the world. I needed her strengths and qualities when I was young and ashamed to be different and afraid my strange other, hidden life would be discovered.

I developed Girl in Life Stream One's qualities to make up for what I feared was my inherent weirdness. Girl in Life Stream One did well. I learned how to navigate the modern world.

Girl One did a good job of protecting Girl Two. Girl Two seems more fragile than Girl One. Maybe that is due to the toll it takes going back and forth between worlds.

I had two lives governed by different rules. Is it possible to be under the auspices of multiple morphic fields, to use Rupert's Sheldrake term? In his book *Dogs That Know When Their Owners are Coming Home* Sheldrake writes of morphic fields, the invisible,

88

overarching guidance systems of social groups of living beings on this planet. These morphic fields

> carry the habitual patterns and "programs" of social organization…. The field is an extended pattern in space-time, just as the gravitational field of the solar system is not merely inside the sun and the planets but contains all of them and coordinates their movements (p. 157).

If you have ever seen a school of fish seeming to explode as each of the fish darts away at the same exact second, you have seen an example of a morphic field in action.

Perhaps these morphic fields extend beyond our world into others, including those our culture views as imaginary. Bryan Appleyard and Holger Kolweit have both commented on the worlds our modern culture no longer give us access to, those populated by beings not of our daily, waking world. Perhaps Girl in Life Stream Two found a way into those worlds. In John Mack's view of reality, these other worlds are termed "third realm." Described by Bryan Appleyard in his remembrance of Mack, "The Aliens Are Always With Us," originally published in the *London Times*, Oct. 3, 2004, "The first realm is that of the mind, the second that of the world, but there is a third realm to which modernity denies us access. And it is there that the aliens live." In this approach, Girl in Life Stream Two is a third-realmer.

Like a cartographer, perhaps I can map that realm to help myself and others.

It is now the day after my birthday, and I am now 55. It has been a few years since I've encountered a mythological beast or a being from a dimension other than ours or become one with subatomic particles around me; however, I continue to slip back and forth in time and hear people speak when they are not actually speaking. My dreams continue to be sources of information and a gateway to other realms. The drives and ambitions of my younger self are mostly played out. I lost who I was in the secret experience-rich years and never really regained that. Girl in Life Stream One, take a bow and then a rest.

I'd like to continue building relationship with the beings or intelligence behind secret experiences. My challenge has been how to move and live in this world in this altered form. This has been true in all areas of my waking life, work, friendships and, most importantly, marriage. I didn't stay single until 47 without becoming well practiced in the art of escape.

I feel I'm now starting to understand how to continue building relationships jointly in my waking world and with whatever is behind my secret experiences. I'm getting an inkling of what it's going to be like to move more consciously between worlds. Maybe we'll run into each other.

# BIBLIOGRAPHY

Anzaldua, Gloria. *Borderlands/La Frontera*. San Francisco: aunt lute books, 1987.

Appleyard, Bryan. "The Aliens Are Always With Us." Originally published in the *London Times*, Oct. 3, 2004; also found on http://johnemackinstitute.org/2004/10/the-aliens-are-always-with-us/)

Atwood, Margaret. *Surfacing*. New York: Doubleday, 1983.

Bolen, Jean Shinoda, *Gods in Everyman*. New York: HarperCollins Publisher, 1989.

Bolen, Jean Shinoda. *Goddesses in Older Women*. New York: HarperCollins Publishers, Inc., 2001.

Bryant, Alice and Linda Seebach, M.S.W. *Healing Shattered Reality: Understanding Contactee Trauma*. Tigard, Oregon: Wildflower Press, 1991.

Donderi, Don, Ph.D. *UFOs, ETs, and Alien Abductions*. Charlottesville, Virginia: Hampton Roads Publishing Company, Inc. 2013.

Eliot, T.S. *Four Quartets*. New York: Harcourt Brace & Company, 1971.

Grof, Christina and Stanislav Grof. *The Stormy Search for the Self*. New York: G.P. Putnam's Sons, 1990.

Heckler, Richard A., Ph.D. *Crossings: Everyday People, Unexpected Events, and Life-Affirming Change*. New York: Harcourt Brace & Company, 1998.

Kolweit, Holder. *Dreamtime and Inner Space: The World of the Shaman*. Boston: Shambhala, 1988.

Lang, Craig R. *The Cosmic Bridge: Close Encounters and Human Destiny*. Morrisville, North Carolina: Lulu Enterprises, Inc., 2007.

ibid. "The More We Learn, the Less We Know. CUFOS International UFO Reporter, 2002.

Keel, John A. *The Complete Guide to Mysterious Beings*. New York: Doubleday, 1994.

Kingsolver, Barbara. *The Poisonwood Bible*. New York: HarperTorch, 1998.

Lessing, Doris. *The Marriages Between Zones Three, Four and Five (as narrated by the Chroniclers of Zone Three).* New York: Alfred A. Knopf, Inc., 1980.

Matheson, Terry. *Alien Abductions: Creating a Modern Phenomenon.* New York: Prometheus Books, 1998.

Miller, George. *Mad Max.* Melbourne, Australia, 1979.

Perera, Sylvia Brinton. *Descent to the Goddess.* Toronto: Inner City Books, 1981.

Sheldrake, Rupert. *Dogs That Know When Their Owners Are Coming Home.* New York: Crown Publishers, 1999.

Strieber, Whitley. *Transformation.* New York: William Morrow, 1988.

"The Sleeping Beauty in the Wood." *The Complete Brothers Grimm Fairy Tales.* New York: Crown Books, 1980.

Vallee, Jacque. *Anatomy of a Phenomenon: Unidentified Objects in Space—A Scientific Appraisal.* Chicago: Henry Regnery Company, 1965.

Ventura, Michael. "A Touch of the Witch." *Twin Cities Reader,* October 1995: 5-6. Print.

Wilber, Ken. *No Boundaries: Eastern and Western Approaches to Personal Growth.* Boston: Shambhala Publications, Inc., 2001

Wilson, Edward O. *Letters to a Young Scientist.* New York: Liveright Publishing Corporation, a division of W. W. Norton & Company, 2013.

Winspear, Jacqueline. *Leaving Everything Most Loved.* New York: Harper Collins Publishers, 2013.

Wolkstein, Diane and Samuel Noah Kramer. *Inanna: Queen of Heaven and Earth.* New York: Harper & Row Publishers, 1983.

# APPENDIX A – SECRET EXPERIENCES DEFINED

This section lists and defines the eight types of secret experiences I've catalogued. I've experienced seven.

List of the eight types of secret experiences:

1. Extraterrestrials / Extradimensionals
2. Physical Invisibility
3. Men in Black
4. Angels
5. Ghosts
6. Children seeing unusual phenomena
7. Giants and demons
8. Endorforms

Definitions of the eight types of secret experiences follow.

## Type 1 – Extraterrestrials / Extradimensionals

I define a Type 1 secret experience as any encounter through any sense with either a being or beings not recognizably human but may appear to have human-like intellect and intention. The experience with these beings may include structures not of our world but in some way are connected to the beings. The encounter may occur during waking or sleep. Changes to the experiencer's feelings, mind and/or body often occur, and these may be moderate or severe. Type 1 secret experiences are typically experienced alone though may occur to multiple members of the same family.

Encounters with or abductions by extraterrestrials are the most commonly-reported type of secret experience. As Bryan Appleyard notes in his article, "The Aliens Are Always With Us," originally published in the *London Times*, Oct. 3, 2004, one estimate is that five million Americans have been abducted by extraterrestrials. His article notes, though, and I paraphrase, we may have gotten the "terrestrial" part wrong and these beings are extradimensionals (for the complete article see http://johnemackinstitute.org/2004/10/the-aliens-are-always-with-us/),

For our purposes we're considering anything "alien" in the category of extraterrestrials and extradimensionals. This allows for a broader interpretation of the beings encountered, and we won't be entering the debate as to what these really are. We'll assume they may be beings either of some planet but just not ours or not at all planet-bound and instead are of the "third realm," a dimension abduction researcher and Harvard psychologist John Mack believed in and explored. Bryan Appleyard writes in "The Aliens Are Always With Us," originally published in the *London Times*, Oct. 3, 2004, "The first realm is that of the mind, the second that of the world, but there is a third realm to which modernity denies us access. And it is there that the aliens live."

## Type 2 - Physical Invisibility

This is defined as periods of time in which a person is not visible to others, and this invisibility may occur spontaneously. The person appears visible to themselves (that is, they can see themselves).

Typically these periods are temporary, and the person once again becomes visible to others.

Some theorize these periods occur around the same time as UFO or extraterrestrial encounters.

Donna Higbie writes on the spontaneous human invisibility phenomena. A good summary of her findings and theories on human invisibility may be found in the article "Spontaneous Human Involuntary Invisibility," which appears in the April 2005 newsletter *The Messenger*, published by the Independent Researchers' Association for Anomalous Phenomena (IRAAP) (article may be found on http://iraap.org/messenger/Messenger8_2.pdf).

## Type 3 – Men in Black

The following information on the Men in Black phenomenon is primarily taken from a personal communication with Dr. Peter M. Rojcewicz in March of 1980 following his talk in Minneapolis on the MIB phenomenon, covered in the *Minneapolis Star Tribune* March 24, 1990.

Peter M. Rocjewicz, Ph.D., Vice President of Academic Affairs and Dean of Faculty at Antioch University, Seattle, as of 2013 and formerly Professor of Mythology at Julliard, writes on the Men in Black or MIB phenomenon and views them as archetypal. In Jungian terms an archetype is a recurring pattern of thought or symbolic imagery derived from the past collective experience and present in the individual unconscious. Archetypes have existence in both myth and the physical world. In Jungian thought they are considered to bridge myth and matter. In this view the appearance of a Man in

Black can both represent a mythical motif as well as a physical presence in our world.

Men in Black encounters often occur after a UFO sighting. In these instances several Men in Black may visit the home of the person who saw the UFO (but didn't necessarily report it) and sometimes will warn against telling anyone else about what they saw. People who have these visits sometimes report the Men in Black seem jerky in speech and movement and often drive a dark, late model car.

Men in Black may also appear solo.

Typically they wear black suits, skinny ties and carry briefcases. Some may sport a bowler.

Men in Black the phenomenon predates *Men in Black* the movie with Will Smith and Tommy Lee Jones.

Rojcewicz says the MIB phenomenon can be traced back to biblical times. He also sees the phenomenon as existing on a continuum: "The Men in Black are part of the extraordinary-encounter continuum—fairies, monsters, ETs, energy forms, flying saucers, flaming crosses," Rojcewicz notes (*Minneapolis Star Tribune*, March 24, 1980).

## Type 4 - Angels

Angels are spiritual beings believed to be separated by one degree from God. While they don't have flesh-and-blood bodies they can materialize in human-like forms with heads and limbs but with the addition of wings. They are often described as being physically beautiful when in their human-like form.

Angels as a tradition exist in both Judaism and Christianity.

They usually have tasks to do in their role as messengers of God and as such are servants to God.

Baruch S. Davidson writes in "What Are Angels" on Chabad.org, "According to Jewish tradition, an angel is a spiritual being and does not have any physical characteristics. The angelic descriptions provided by the prophets – such as wings, arms etc. – are anthropomorphic, referring to their spiritual abilities and tasks" (http://www.chabad.org/library/article_cdo/aid/692875/jewish/What-Are-Angels.htm ).

Guardian angels are assigned to specific humans to guide and protect.

Anecdotally, more people report seeing and being aware of guardian angels than seeing "regular" angels. However, there are reports of people hearing "regular" angels.

Paulette Salo, known as the angel artist, sees individuals' guardian angels and will paint the guardian angel's portrait as a keepsake for the individual so they may see and speak to their angel (for complete details see http://www.angelsbypaulette.com ).

## Type 5 - Ghosts

I'm defining ghosts as humans who have physically died but continue to manifest in some way in our physical dimension. Theories abound as to why ghosts "haunt" certain locations. Most common is the theory that they have unfinished business. Ghosts include poltergeists. Literally "noisy spirit," poltergeists commonly cause noises and objects to move around. More recently, those who investigate such things lean toward a definition that claims the activity emanates from the unconscious mind of individuals involved in the manifestation, usually those on the cusp of puberty. Ghosts are the only secret experience I haven't had (that I'm aware of). We had lights turning off and on in our lower level when all of my family was of an age to be living at home and, once, objects unpacking themselves from deep storage in a building on my parents' property. I'd called my mom to request that she send my black patent leather tap shoes for an art installation in graduate school. She went to the storage building to find them, and, as she climbed the steps to the upper level, was greeted by the tap shoes sitting expectantly on the top step.

Type 6 - Children seeing unusual phenomena

Anecdotally, it seems the types of phenomenon children encounter are the same as those encountered by adults; however, children may have different responses to the encounter. Here I'm using the biological definition of "child," anyone between the stages of birth and puberty. Technically I was a child when my secret experiences started though my response to those early encounters—rides around the universe with "Eric" in a Jetson-style spaceship—left me awakening as though from a nightmare, wild-eyed with fright and fear. However, at least one person, Bob, has reported to me that a child he knows has observed the ghost of her dead father apparently without shock or fear.

## Type 7 - Giants and demons

Giants are considered to be monsters with human-like characteristics but of colossal size and strength.

In my experience they were of colossal size and of human shape but entirely covered in bronze. The particular one I saw on the road to Smithfield, Virginia, one morning on the way to work, was stationary, as though he'd accidently stepped into our dimension and was trying to figure out where he was.

Demons are often considered to be fallen angels, evil, intent on wreaking havoc and sometimes under the power of another. As fallen angels, their original beauty is twisted into malign features, and they are often portrayed as small in stature.

Alice Bryant and Linda Seebach in their book *Healing Shattered Reality* include "nightmares or dreams of strange beings and other worlds" in a list of experiences that may indicate a person is a contactee of "Dimension Travelers" or extraterrestrials (p. 7; Author's Forward). The giant and the demon I saw were strange beings, but I saw them during waking time, not during a dream, so my experiences don't fit Bryant and Seebach's criteria. However, yours might, so I include the possibility that seeing or encountering giants and/or demons may stand for something else.

## Type 8 - Endorforms

Endoforms are "forms within forms." I include them here because of my one experience with a being within me that called itself an endoform when I asked what it was. At the time I assumed I was the form hosting the form. I understood it to be male. After several months of being in residence within me one particular night its voice grew glorious and full of excitement. The next day I learned a coworker and friend had given birth to a baby boy the night before. Was I hearing the voice of her baby boy all those months when she was the host, not me?

# APPENDIX B – SECRET EXPERIENCES MATRIX: FEELINGS AND RESPONSES

The eight secret experiences run across the top, the feelings and responses along the side.

| | Extraterrestrials or extradimensionals | Invisibility | Men in Black | Ghosts | Angels | Children's secret experiences | Giants and demons | Endoforms |
|---|---|---|---|---|---|---|---|---|
| Interrupted sleep | X | | X | | | X | | |
| Extreme fright[2] | X | | X | | | X | X | |
| Questioning whether it really happened | X | X | X | X | X | | X | |
| Ontological shock / feeling you're coming apart | X | X | X | | | | X | |
| Feel hunted | X | | | | | | | |
| Desire to be on the move | X | X | X | | | | X | X |
| Replaying the experience in thoughts | X | X | X | | | | | |

---

[2] Includes feeling paralyzed and unable to move.

Matrix, continued:

| | Extraterrestrials or extradimensionals | Invisibility | Men in Black | Ghosts | Angels | Children's secret experiences | Giants and demons | Endoforms |
|---|---|---|---|---|---|---|---|---|
| Development of an internal red-alert system | X | | | | | | | |
| Physical anomalies | X | X | X | | | | X | |
| Emotional pattern development | | | | | | | | |
| Wonder | X | | | X | X | X | | |
| Exhilaration | | | | | X | | | |
| Awe | X | | | | X | | | |
| Wonder | X | | | X | X | | | X |
| Curiosity | | | | | | X | | X |
| Connection | X | | | X | | | | X |
| Adapting | X | | | | | | | |
| Developing relationship with intelligence behind SEs | X | | | | | | | |

# ABOUT THE AUTHOR

Karen Cavalli is the author of fiction and non-fiction, and her work appears online and in print books and magazines. Her writing has won awards including Outstanding Secondary Science Book. She has written and taught on anomalous experiences. She writes and lives near Minneapolis, Minnesota, with her husband. Visit www.karencavalli.com

www.ingramcontent.com/pod-product-compliance
Lightning Source LLC
Chambersburg PA
CBHW060415290526
45791CB00002B/767